# Ethel Gordon Fenwick

# Ethel Gordon Fenwick

## Nursing Reformer and the First Registered Nurse

Jenny Main

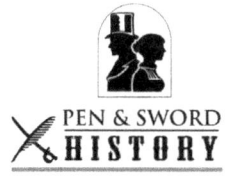

First published in Great Britain in 2022 by
Pen & Sword History
An imprint of
Pen & Sword Books Ltd
Yorkshire – Philadelphia

Copyright © Jenny Main 2022

ISBN 978 1 39909 958 5

The right of Jenny Main to be identified as Author of this work has been asserted by her in accordance with the Copyright, Designs and Patents Act 1988.

A CIP catalogue record for this book is available from the British Library.

All rights reserved. No part of this book may be reproduced or transmitted in any form or by any means, electronic or mechanical including photocopying, recording or by any information storage and retrieval system, without permission from the Publisher in writing.

Typeset by Mac Style
Printed and bound in the UK by CPI Group (UK) Ltd, Croydon, CR0 4YY.

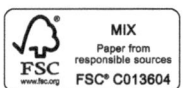

Pen & Sword Books Limited incorporates the imprints of Atlas, Archaeology, Aviation, Discovery, Family History, Fiction, History, Maritime, Military, Military Classics, Politics, Select, Transport, True Crime, Air World, Frontline Publishing, Leo Cooper, Remember When, Seaforth Publishing, The Praetorian Press, Wharncliffe Local History, Wharncliffe Transport, Wharncliffe True Crime and White Owl.

For a complete list of Pen & Sword titles please contact

PEN & SWORD BOOKS LIMITED
47 Church Street, Barnsley, South Yorkshire, S70 2AS, England
E-mail: enquiries@pen-and-sword.co.uk
Website: www.pen-and-sword.co.uk

Or

PEN AND SWORD BOOKS
1950 Lawrence Rd, Havertown, PA 19083, USA
E-mail: Uspen-and-sword@casematepublishers.com
Website: www.penandswordbooks.com

# Contents

| | | |
|---|---|---|
| *Introduction* | | vi |
| **Chapter 1** | The Foundations: 1857–1877 | 1 |
| **Chapter 2** | Women, Work, Medicine, and Nursing up to the 1870s | 19 |
| **Chapter 3** | Old Medicine, the New Nurse, and Promotion: 1878–1897 | 34 |
| **Chapter 4** | The Matron 1881–1887 | 49 |
| **Chapter 5** | Celebrations, Marriage, and New Challenges 1887–1899 | 70 |
| **Chapter 6** | The New Era: Some Success 1900–1909 | 98 |
| **Chapter 7** | Battles, Deaths, and Victories 1910–1919 | 122 |
| **Chapter 8** | Registration and Professionalism 1919–1946 | 151 |
| *Acknowledgements* | | 180 |
| *Sources* | | 182 |
| *Index* | | 183 |

# Introduction

'Mrs. Bedford Fenwick was a woman with whom it was possible to do business on terms of complete subservience.'

So wrote Lord Inman in his autobiography. A medical colleague of Ethel, Harrison Cripps FRCS, described her as a 'restless genius', which raises the question – what went into the making of such an awe-inspiring character and what sort of world did she live in?

Today, very few people know anything about the remarkable Ethel Gordon Fenwick, who worked so hard for the benefit of nurses and, ultimately, their patients. She was instrumental in forming a respected profession out of what had been several dedicated, but disparate and unregulated, groups of women. Regardless of skill, experience, or competence, before 1920, anyone could call themselves a nurse. With extraordinary foresight, Ethel Fenwick saw the need for properly trained nurses to organise and protect their professional interests and for almost thirty years she led them in the battle for professional registration.

Born Ethel Gordon Manson, she lived at a time of immense political and social changes, when the foundations of modern medicine were being formed. She was born into a world that had no lightbulbs or telephones, where transport was by horseback, carts, carriages, ships, and early steam trains. In her last years, she saw electricity in most homes, the internal combustion engine replacing the horse, and the jet engine and Spitfire obtaining mastery of the skies.

When Ethel was in her infancy, medicine was primitive, and nursing was only just beginning to be appreciated as a skilled occupation. At the age of 21, when she went to work in the Children's Hospital

Nottingham, she was described as 'full of spirit, with a will of steel' and these characteristics were to prove essential throughout her life of campaigning. She obtained the prestigious post of matron of St Bartholomew's hospital at the extraordinarily young age of 24, and during her six years of hard work there she instigated improvements in conditions for both staff and patients. She introduced reforms in nursing and won the respect of older established sisters and medical staff – one being Harrison Cripps FRCS, the colleague who described her as a 'restless genius'.

When she married, Ethel was obliged to leave her hospital work but, as Mrs Ethel Bedford Fenwick, she continued her work to create a recognised and registered profession of nursing. Although Queen Victoria did not approve, Ethel gained the support of royalty in her campaign to improve nursing standards and, despite their differing opinions, Ethel built upon the foundations laid by Florence Nightingale. She was also influenced by the innovative American nurses she met on her travels and with whom she shared friendship, ideals, and objectives within the fields of nursing and of female emancipation.

The key to creating the professional status of nursing was the education of nurses, and a consistent standard for a training curriculum throughout Britain was essential. In insisting on national standards of the highest level, Ethel ensured that, having qualified by passing a professional examination, a nurse could be registered as part of a well-regulated professional organisation with the right to be responsible for, and to direct, their own field of expertise.

Since her day, the worlds of nursing and medicine have changed almost beyond recognition. In the 1960s, nurses were still obliged to live in the nurses' home, supervised by a Home Sister for the first two years of their training. As the workforce of the hospital wards, they were taught as they worked alongside senior and trained nurses. Weeks of lectures in the training school were interspersed with the 'hands on' ward placements during the students' three-year training. At the end of each ward placement, the Ward Sister would sign every successfully completed procedure in the student nurse's precious booklet of achievements. Pay for a first-year student nurse in 1967 was £365 a year, with £143 deducted for board and lodging, and male nurses were a rarity. After registration, a qualified Staff Nurse was paid £690 a year.

Changes in uniform have been slow but inexorable. Up until the 1970s, nurses in mufti could be identified by the angry red marks caused by the rubbing of the solidly starched cuffs and collars on their soft skin. Once, nurses would obsessively check every starched fold, crease, and ribbon of their uniforms when these were returned from the hospital laundry. Later, ribbonless caps were attached as if by magic, it being a matter of pride that no hair grip was ever revealed. Nowadays, being abandoned altogether, unstable headwear no longer causes anxiety and crisply starched aprons have been replaced by disposable plastic worn over practical trousers and tunics.

Linseed poultices and starched aprons have now given way to antibiotics and disposable gloves. Vanquished from the modern ward sluice of today are the racks of metal bedpans and the rails of carefully hand-washed cotton bandages of all sizes, including the 'many-tailed' abdominal bandage. Junior nurses no longer escape from a demanding Ward Sister by hiding in the relative sanctuary of the sluice room to wash endless rubber sheets in the massive sinks. Ward cupboards that once housed Nelson inhalers, mercury thermometers, enamel basins, gum catheters, rubber tubing, jugs, funnels, and buckets nowadays contain endless packets of disposable dressings, single-use equipment and complex electronic devices.

In spite of modern advances, many old nursing traditions persist, even if their original purpose is forgotten – such as pillowcase openings facing away from the door. Supposedly originating in the days of Florence Nightingale and the Crimea, this practice was in order to keep the pervasive sand from blowing inside the pillow. Reminiscent of bloody bandages, red and white flowers in the same vase remain strictly taboo, being considered an invitation for an unpredicted visit from the Grim Reaper.

The development of scientific methods of anaesthesia and of antisepsis provided a new role for the nurse and in 1973 Winifred Hector, Sister Tutor of St Bartholomew's, wrote:

> It is only in the eighteenth century that we begin to see the emergence of ward life as we recognise it, and in the nineteenth that we see our predecessors and the role of the modern nurse begin to shape itself; while in the last hundred years we have a well-documented account of the rapid evolution of the professional nurse as we know her today.

Ethel Fenwick saw several wars with their inherent horrors, and made major contributions in organising the nursing of soldiers in theatres of war in Greece and France, where her expertise was invaluable. For her efforts, she received several medals acknowledging her work, including:

- Silver French medal engraved: *Ministere de la Sante Publique – Assistance – Mrs. Bedford Fenwick 1933*
- Medaille Reconnaissance Francaise 1921
- Primrose league medal
- King George and Queen Mary Silver Jubilee medal
- British College of Nurses silver medal
- British College of Nurses gold medal, presented 1928
- Royal British Nurse Association medals, one enamelled, one bronze

These medals were eventually donated to the St Bartholomew's hospital archives by her grandson, David, who remembered her with pride, affection, and not a little awe. It is claimed that she turned down other awards that were offered by the British establishment.

Ethel was very aware of the danger of nurses looking inward within their profession, and, as editor of the *British Journal of Nursing*, did her best to expand horizons by constantly exploring wider world issues. As an ardent Suffragist, she recognised early on that, without the right to vote, women and nurses were powerless to affect developments within their country or within their profession. She enjoyed writing and editing, continuing the work for fifty-three years, almost until her death. The *British Journal of Nursing* was distributed in all English-speaking countries and, as editor and frequent contributor, she was an influence for professional nursing organisations in many countries. Her journal survived her by nine years.

Ethel Fenwick's other great achievement was the creation of the International Congress of Nurses, having developed the idea from meetings of the International Council of Women. With her abilities as orator and journalist, she inspired a generation of nurses to realise their part in the progress of international peace.

While Ethel was an inspiring and determined leader, her unyielding adherence to her principles made her a poor politician. The moderating influence of her colleague and friend Isla Stewart was invaluable but, after Isla's death in 1910, Ethel became more autocratic and, as a result, was eventually isolated from the mainstream of the nursing movement. It must not be forgotten that, without her determination and fighting spirit during the many hard-fought years, the cause of registration would not have advanced as successfully as it did.

Even her opponents admired her strength of character and her tenacity – vital qualities in an age before women were allowed to vote and when a patriarchal establishment had total control. Ethel did not believe a nurse was merely a servant of the doctor, but should be valued as a competent colleague. Thanks to her foresight and dogged determination over many hard-fought years, qualified nurses were organised and ready, after the second World War, to take their place alongside other professions within the newly formed Health Service.

In 1999, the Royal College of Nursing hosted the Centennial Conference of the International Council of Nurses in London and in the run up to this event a commemorative plaque to Ethel was unveiled at 20, Upper Wimpole Street. The wording on the plaque reads:

Ethel Gordon Fenwick
1857–1947
Nursing Reformer
lived here
1887–1924

Ethel Gordon Fenwick is deservedly the first name on the list of Registered Nurses. The following chapters reveal a little of the many innovations, scientific discoveries, and social changes which influenced her years and which have shaped our world today.

# Chapter 1

# The Foundations: 1857–1877

Ethel Gordon Manson was born into a Victorian world and she was to see many changes throughout her lifetime. When she was born, transport was mostly horse-drawn, with new-fangled steam engines beginning to make their mark. Having lived through two World Wars, she died ninety years later – just as the new National Health Service Act was making its way through Parliament.

The 1851 census records her father: 'David Manson, Spynie House, aged 40, widower, physician but not practicing at the time, farmer.' Scotsman David Manson came from Croy near Inverness, his mother being from a collateral branch of the Rose family of Kilravock. After training in Edinburgh, he qualified as a doctor sometime around 1831 but did not practice medicine. He married an American heiress, Kezia Scott, whose family had returned to Scotland after losing a fortune in the American Civil War. On the death of his brother, David had inherited Spynie Farm, in the nearby county of Moray, becoming responsible for employing eleven labourers, nine women, and three house servants. In 1846, his wife Kezia died in her early thirties, a not uncommon occurrence in those times when childbirth was a dangerous business and when there were no antibiotics to treat the many diseases common at that time. Kezia was buried in Spynie churchyard.

Once an important part of Pictish territory, Spynie lies in the north-east corner of Scotland, two miles north from the county town of Elgin. Many centuries ago, the sea drove far inland and the River Lossie poured into a great five-mile-wide estuary, eventually forming a great sea loch. In 1040 the last Pictish Mormaer, (King) Macbeth, slew his rival, King Duncan, at Pitgaveny, which adjoins Spynie. By the nineteenth century, fishing villages lined the edges of the large sea loch, overlooked by the great building of the Bishop's Palace. There was a busy salt industry and ships would berth in a small harbour below Spynie ridge, which was, at that time, the port for the town of Elgin.

Throughout its colourful past, Spynie Palace has been visited by many famous figures, not least the much-travelled Mary, Queen of Scots. Following the completion of Elgin Cathedral in 1224, a variety of bishops lived in Spynie Palace, including Bishop David Stewart who was responsible for building the massive tower in the fifteenth century. The last bishop, Patrick Hepburn, died there, debauched and dissolute, in 1573. Seventeenth-century storms changed the mouth of the river and the landscape of the estuary, causing the waters of the loch to recede. Enterprising landowners began to drain the land, Thomas Telford drew up plans for a canal network and, despite setbacks caused by more storms and floods, by the end of the nineteenth century, land had been reclaimed for agriculture. A railway line was built across what had once been the great Spynie Loch, with trains running the five miles from Elgin past the ruins of the Bishop's Palace of Spynie on to the nearest harbour at Lossiemouth.

Nowadays, all that remains of the great body of water is Spynie Loch wildlife reserve, visited, as it has been for millennia, by great flocks of geese during the winter and where a wide variety of birds nest in the sheltering reed beds. The defunct railway track runs between the loch and the palace, and the semi-restored palace ruins are now in the care of Historic Scotland. Looking north from the top of the palace tower, the hills of Easter Ross and Sutherland can clearly be seen across the waters of the Moray Firth. Visible beyond the town of Elgin, the bulk of Ben Rinnes, outlier of the distant Cairngorm mountains, overlooks the fertile Laich of Moray, through which the two great salmon rivers, the Spey and the Lossie, rush to the sea.

The area has played a part in history and seen its fair share of politics, battles, and skirmishes, but what was once a scene full of bustling activity is now a peaceful agricultural landscape. The role of

Spynie Farm has changed since the early days of supplying food for the medieval bishops. The foundations of the original Spynie parish church, built beside the palace, are barely visible but the graveyard remains and contains amongst others, the final resting place of Kezia Manson and, later, Ramsay MacDonald. A new Church of Spynie was completed in 1736 at nearby Quarrywood and incorporated the original old Spynie Church bell.

When he was in his early forties, David Manson, living in the relatively modern establishment of Spynie House, married again, this time a Yorkshire lass, Harriette Palmer of Thurnscoe. David and Harriette had two daughters, firstly Clara, and then Ethel two years later. This second daughter, Ethel Gordon Manson, born in January 1857, was to become one of the most tenacious nursing reformers of her day. Because a child from David's first marriage had married a Gordon, Ethel was given this as a middle name when her birth was registered by her half-brother.

Gordon is a name of great antiquity and with a long history in Moray. Seat of the Dukes of Gordon, Gordon Castle lies beside the mighty river Spey, ten miles from Elgin, and the building was once over quarter of a mile in length. Over centuries of battles and war, the powerful Gordon clan had a great influence in and beyond Moray; generations of the Dukes of Richmond and Gordon and their families playing a great part in politics and also in both Scottish and English high society. Once indicative of clan membership, the name has nowadays also been used as a forename, but can often still indicate a clan connection. The first Highland Games of the season are now held annually at Gordon Castle and the great walled garden still nurtures some beautiful, productive and ancient fruit trees. Modern cuisine with produce from the estate and garden is nowadays served in a popular restaurant, a restored estate building, beside the walled garden. The estate now produces a selection of popular herbal and plant-based products, including a specialist gin.

Ethel was just nine months old when, in September 1857, at the age of 46, her father David Manson died of heart failure, leaving his wife

Harriette pregnant with their son. Before his little daughter Ethel had taken her first steps, David was buried beside his first wife in Spynie churchyard. His son Eric was born at Spynie a few weeks later on 12 December 1857.

Throughout Britain, this was a time of massive social upheaval with wide disruptions and changes in agriculture and industry. Scotland had been left disrupted for years following the aftermath of Culloden in 1745 and the clan system had been effectively destroyed. Vast areas of the country were left barren and empty after several famines had been followed by the iniquitous Land Clearances, with the destruction of communities continuing until 1860. Many Scots had been forced to seek a new life in countries overseas and, with the influx of the dispossessed and the adventurous, these young communities in the New World were developing rapidly.

Victorians were building their great Empire and entrepreneurs were amassing enormous fortunes. Men of intellect were busily observing, recording, arguing, and postulating their favourite theories, trying to create order from the perceived chaos of nature. Inventors were attempting to translate ideas into action, new efforts were being made to communicate across distances, and new machines were designed to travel more efficiently and to explore every environment.

In Great Britain, women's suffrage was demanded by the Chartist movement of the 1840s, having been first advocated by Mary Wollstonecraft in her book *A Vindication of the Rights of Woman* in 1792. (Her daughter, Mary, married the poet Shelley, and wrote the chilling novel *Frankenstein* in 1818.) The call for women's suffrage was increasingly taken up by liberal intellectuals from the 1850s onwards, notably by the philosopher, writer, social reformer, and eventual Member of Parliament, John Stuart Mill, and his wife, Harriet.

All was not peaceful in the great British Empire. A revolt by Indian sepoys in the East India Company's Bengal army at Meerut grew into a full-scale uprising, resulting in the Indian Mutiny in 1857. This rebellion was savagely suppressed, but it marked the end of a century of government by the East India Company, which was then replaced by a Viceroy governing in the name of Queen Victoria.

Queen Victoria's eldest daughter, the Princess Royal, married Prince Frederick William of Prussia and two years later, in January 1859, gave birth to the Prince destined to become Emperor Wilhelm II – the man later to be known as the Kaiser.

The first half of the nineteenth century had been a time of great religious debate and revival. Sunday was strictly observed, new churches had been built, with many disparate and often contentious church groups being formed. However, with the economic boom in Britain between 1850 and the 1870s, many from the rural population moved into the towns looking for work and eventually religion began to play less and less of a part in their lives. In spite of the efforts of revival crusades, church attendances began to fall. The equilibrium of society was shaken in 1859 when, after much agonising, Darwin published his book *On the Origin of Species*. This revolutionary theory, suggesting natural selection and survival of the fittest, was a direct challenge to the previously unquestioned belief that, a mere few thousand years earlier, God had created every living thing in its final form.

Concerning more domestic matters, young Isabella Beeton published the first instalment of her book on household management, which was to become a classic reference book. As well as cooking instructions and recipes, she also gave advice about instructing the eighteen grades of servant found in an ideal household establishment, with guidelines on etiquette and economy. She died a few short years later, at the young age of 28, during her fourth confinement. Childbirth was a dangerous and frequently fatal undertaking in those days.

In 1859, Charles Dickens published *A Tale of Two Cities*, and John Stuart Mill published *On Liberty*. Within a few months Florence Nightingale published *Notes on Nursing: What It Is, and What It Is Not*, which was to become an essential guide to the progressive improvements in nursing skills. Inspired by the example of her work, and after witnessing the horrors of the Battle of Solferino, Henri Dunant founded the Red Cross and brought about the Geneva Convention of 1864.

Patent medicines were much in vogue at the time, one being the strange oil which was discovered seeping from the ground in places such as Pennsylvania, USA. The oil was blotted up with blankets and used to cure anything from scrofula to diarrhoea. A self-styled colonel, retired railway porter Edwin Drake, was convinced that the oil could be retrieved from the ground by wells. In 1859, he bored down 69ft, achieved the world's first gusher and, in three months, Titusville, Pennsylvania sprung from nothing into a town with a population of 15,000 hopeful entrepreneurs. Unimaginable industrial changes lay ahead.

Determined to liberate America's slaves and set up a new nation in north-western Virginia, John Brown and his twenty-one supporters captured the Harpers Ferry federal armoury which contained 100,000 rifles and ammunition. He was hanged for his temerity a month later, consequently turned into a martyr and celebrated in song. Southern loyalists rose up in arms and soon the young American nation was at war with itself. The first shot in the American Civil War was fired on 9 January 1861. Because of this war, the cotton-growing industry collapsed and more than half a million British Lancashire cotton industry workers were deprived of work and wages. As a direct consequence, cotton cultivation was encouraged in India. Britain remained strictly neutral in the American Civil War although, following an incident where an American steamer stopped a British steamship in the Bahamas, the risk of war between the two countries was very real for a time.

When Ethel Gordon Manson was still a toddler, her mother married again in 1859 and took her young children – Clara, Ethel, and Eric – to their new home at Thoroton in the Vale of Belvoir, Nottinghamshire, owned by her new husband, George Storer. Mentioned in the Doomsday book, Thoroton lies on the west bank of the river Smite and is fifteen miles east from the city of Nottingham, with the Roman road – the Fosse Way – three miles to the east.

Made of red brick, double-ranged, Thoroton Hall has two storeys and garrets, and was built in the early eighteenth century on the site of an earlier building. Improvements and alterations were carried out in the early nineteenth century when kitchen and service wings were added. Oak beams in one of the rooms are thought to have come from the earlier timber-framed manor house. Stone flagged entrance hall, oak panelling, doors with brass fitments, sashed windows, window shutters and splendid eighteenth-century fire-grates in most of the bedrooms all gave character to the house. A boundary wall surrounded the property, which contained several brick-built outbuildings including stables, a small forge, and a bakehouse. The substantial garden, surrounded by impressive trees, provided plenty of space for the children to explore and play.

The property was passed on to George Storer through his mother and the census of 1851 lists him as aged 36, living there as head of the household with a cook, a housemaid, a groom, and one farmworker. George Storer had been educated at Louth Grammar School and at St. John's College Cambridge and by then was a gentleman farmer, overseeing 431 acres with the assistance of six labourers and a young boy. He had a special interest in rearing Shorthorn cattle and held the directorship of the Shorthorn Dairy Company Ltd. He was a keen foxhunter, participating in hunt meetings alongside the Duke of Rutland, and was a Justice of the Peace at the Bingham Petty sessions and the Notts Epiphany Quarter sessions. He was also a captain in the 2nd Leicestershire (Belvoir) Rifles and, conventionally, when aged over forty, it was about time he had a wife.

In an era when women relied on men for support, Ethel's mother Harriette was in need of a husband and a home of her own. She was experienced with farm and country living and was more than capable of running a large household. She was a tall, imposing woman whose striking appearance was in keeping with her strength of character and she was very aware that she came from a proud and distinguished family. (In her later years the family referred to her privately as 'the Grenadier'!)

In complete contrast, Ethel's stepfather, George Storer, was a small man and privately known in the family as 'the widow's mite'. He was to prove a kindly influence on Ethel and she was fortunate to grow up in an environment that encouraged her interest in the rapidly developing world and the expanding British Empire. Harriette and her children soon settled into their new home in an arrangement that suited them all.

The 1860s saw the era of the train and the development of communications; railways being built with the telegraph system often running alongside railway lines. By the time Abraham Lincoln became American President in March 1861, the Morse telegraph system was operating nationwide in the United States.

In Britain the abolition of stamp duty on paper resulted in the expansion of Sunday papers. The collection of information, especially from Reuter's London headquarters, revolutionised journalism and the distribution of news. Coincidentally, and fortuitously, the fine delicacy known as fish and chips was introduced to the British public palate around the same time. In the British countryside, ploughing engines designed by Wiltshire man John Fowler were making an appearance, although the self-propelled engines caused problems due to their weight on the poor roads. Local authorities and landowners restricted movements of these great new machines, but this did not deter innovators such as Thomas Aveling, who designed and built the forerunner of the mighty traction engine.

Queen Victoria was devastated and Britain was plunged into mourning when, as a direct consequence of the bad drains at Windsor Castle, Prince Albert died of typhoid fever on 15 December 1861. Never physically robust, Albert had become increasingly unwell after catching a chill, and the worry over the deterioration in relations between America and Great Britain increased the burden on his health. Although desperately ill, on 1 December, when hostilities seemed likely, he drafted a memorandum with amendments for the Queen to put in her draft dispatches. This undoubtedly helped avert a crisis between the two governments of America and Great Britain at a time when they were on the verge of war. However, even royalty was not able to control the ravages of disease and, as his condition worsened and he became delirious, Victoria could only watch helplessly. Albert's death caused nationwide shock and sorrow and the Queen was consumed in grief.

During Ethel's childhood, the cotton famine brought starvation and disaster to mill workers in Lancashire. The first section of the world's first underground railway, the Metropolitan Railway Line from Paddington to Farringdon Street, was opened in 1863. Troubles in Ireland caused much debate in Parliament, and Broadmoor Asylum for the criminally insane was established in Berkshire. Child welfare was a matter for some concern and Acts of Parliament were passed to prevent persons under 16 years of age from engaging in sweeping, cleaning or coring a chimney or flue. Small children would no longer be sent up chimneys and risk becoming lost or stuck while attempting to clear them. The science of modern metallurgy was born when Henry Clifton Sorby discovered the micro-structure of steel, and in the same year the Swedish chemist, Alfred Nobel, patented a mixture of nitroglycerine and gunpowder.

The British Prime Minister, Lord Palmerston, died and was succeeded by Lord John Russell, with William Gladstone becoming Leader of the House. A year later, Octavia Hill began a campaign to reform slum housing in London. William Booth founded the East London Christian Mission in Whitechapel, London, in 1865.

As the British Empire expanded, traders and whalers took their alien customs and devastating diseases to the islands of the South Pacific, causing increasing disruption to the traditional ways of life. Settlers in New Zealand fought bitter territorial battles with the native Māori. In Jamaica, a black uprising resulted in martial law being declared, followed by excessive repression, punishments, and the execution of the leaders of the uprising. The first transatlantic telegraph cable was laid in 1865 and, in April that year, Americans were stunned by the assassination of President Lincoln.

In London, in July 1865, James Barry died. Only then was it discovered that this 'most skillful of physicians and most wayward of men' was in reality a woman and had possibly born a child. A medical career was impossible for a woman in those days, but 'James' Miranda Stuart Barry, born in 1790, had graduated from Edinburgh University, joined the British Army and practiced medicine for fifty-two years. Successfully disguised as a man, she served in the Cape of Good Hope, Mauritius, Jamaica, St Helena, and Corfu, where she treated casualties of the Crimea. During her service, Dr Barry worked her way up from surgeon's mate until, in 1857, she became Inspector-General of Military Hospitals in Montreal and Quebec.

Alfred Nobel, still experimenting with explosive mixtures, patented dynamite in 1866, after demonstrating its action at a quarry at Redhill. Thomas Aveling had produced a road roller driven by steam, but the 1865 Locomotive Act severely restricted operations and the imposition of a speed limit of 2mph in towns and 4mph in the country, with regulations requiring a man to walk in front of the machine with warning red flag, held back development. Understandably, railways expanded rapidly as the road system stagnated. However, the machines were exported to places such as eastern Europe where higher speeds were allowed and the engines were converted for straw burning. Ploughing engines were exported to Egypt and the road steamer helped open up remote territories such as those in India.

Irishman Thomas Barnardo founded the East End Mission for destitute children in 1866 in Stepney and this was followed by several other London homes which became known as the Dr Barnardo Homes. A cholera epidemic ravaged Britain in 1866 while, a couple of miles from Ethel's birthplace, future Prime Minister Ramsay MacDonald was born. Nelson's column was unveiled in Trafalgar Square and the foundation of the Albert Hall was laid.

In America, following the Civil War, the US Congress passed the Civil Rights Act of 1866, which finally gave full citizenship rights to black Americans. The Dominion of Canada was formed in 1867 and the government there was given almost sovereign powers.

British farmers suffered from a poor harvest and, although the Continent was worse affected, cattle plague entered Britain and a licence was required to move any cattle. Society was restless; there were riots in Hyde Park and the Irish Fenian conspiracy resulted in the suspension of the *Habeaus Corpus* law in Ireland. The 1867 Clerkenwell explosion resulted in several people being killed but failed in the objective of freeing Fenian prisoners. Also, in 1867 the contentious *Das Kapital* by Karl Marx was published.

The first women's suffrage committee had been formed in Manchester in 1865, and in 1867 John Stuart Mill presented their petition to Parliament. The petition, containing about 1,550 signatures, demanded the vote for women. It was to be a long hard struggle, with many more petitions and millions more signatures, before women's suffrage was achieved in Britain.

The surgeon Joseph Lister used the technique of covering open wounds with dressing soaked in carbolic acid (phenol) and performed the first operation under antiseptic conditions at Glasgow Infirmary. His experiments with hand washing, sterilising instruments, and spraying carbolic acid in the theatre while operating succeeded in lowering the infection rate. From then on, surgical procedures became less deadly. The last public execution in Britain took place outside Newgate prison in 1868, the hanged man having been convicted of murdering twelve people with a bomb.

The transcontinental rail link across America was completed in 1869 when the Central Pacific and Union Pacific joined tracks at Utah. By this time, several different British railway companies were finding themselves in financial difficulties. Between 1867 and 1873, a Wisconsin man, Christopher Latham Sholes, worked to develop the typewriter – a machine that would change the workplace, the world, and the lives of many women.

Social reform was in the air, the abuses of the gang system of labour as well as the evils of child labourers were debated in Parliament and it was proposed to give suffrage to urban labourers. The Reform Bill of 1867 contained no provision for women's suffrage, but suffrage societies were forming in most of the major cities of Britain. By the 1870s, these organisations submitted to Parliament petitions containing a total of almost three million signatures demanding the franchise for women.

Before the 1868 General Election, 80 per cent of food was home produced, but then farming went into a depression. As a result of the mechanisation of farming methods, thousands of people had moved out of the countryside and into towns to seek jobs. Along with the increase in mechanisation and industrialisation came the increase of slums and poverty. The dreaded workhouse provided shelter of a sort for the desperately destitute, but their overcrowded and insanitary conditions also provided an ideal breeding ground for disease.

Back in Ethel's home county of Moray, in 1868, entrepreneur George Baxter gave up his work as a gardener at Gordon Castle, Fochabers, and opened a little grocery shop. His wife Margaret made her jams and jellies in the back of the shop and, slowly but surely, a thriving local industry was born which, was eventually to supply top quality produce to high-class establishments and shops throughout Britain for generations.

By 1869, communications between Britain and India were revolutionised with the opening of the Suez Canal, while the British Empire continued its relentless march across the globe – annexing the Kimberly diamond mines in South Africa.

The first university college for women, later named Girton College, was founded at Cambridge in 1869 and that same year the Education Act instigated compulsory primary education in Britain. The Married Women's Property Act extended the rights of women to own property in marriage, although many restrictions remained.

George Storer, Ethel's stepfather, was instrumental in establishing a Chamber of Agriculture for Nottinghamshire in 1869 and became their first president. He was also a key member of the Notts branch of the

National Union of Conservative and Constitutional Association. The census of 1871 records George Storer, 56, as head of the household, a magistrate, farmer of 420 acres, now employing eleven farm workers and four boys. By that time Harriette, his wife, was aged 40, his stepdaughter Clara was 16 and Ethel was 14.

At the beginning of the Victorian age, while Ethel was growing into a young woman, the population of Britain was around 15 million, but before the end of the century it had reached 37 million. By 1870, when Charles Dickens died, more than 60 per cent of people in Britain were literate. The 1870 Education Act, which required compulsory primary education, and the subsequent expansion of schools, resulted in more than 95 per cent of the population being able to read and write by end of the century.

As was the custom, the young children of Thoroton Hall were educated at home. When Ethel and her sister were old enough, they were sent to Middlethorpe Hall, near York, to be educated privately at the girls' boarding school, which took in young ladies from the ages of 9–18. Middlethorpe had been leased out by Dr Matthew Wilkinson, a much-respected Manchester physician who had trained in Edinburgh. One of the pupils at the school, two years older than Ethel, was his daughter Fanny who, after overcoming many objections and obstacles, was to become Britain's first female landscape horticulturalist.

Growing up in a house with plenty of domestic staff, Ethel soon developed the abilities to organise and supervise whilst absorbing an appreciation of fine antiques, furniture, books and clothes. She was fortunate to enter her formative teenage years in a school where she met pupils from progressive thinking families. Living in a politically aware household, her interest in world affairs was encouraged and she developed a keen interest in the news and the issues of the times.

In 1870, the American Congress passed the Fifteenth Amendment, which required all southern states to allow blacks to vote and, as a result of this Amendment, Thomas Peterson-Mundy became the first black man to cast a vote in an election. Meanwhile, scientists developed some strange theories in attempts to justify popular prejudice, and it was postulated that non-Caucasian and also female brains were inferior in size and quality.

From the 1870s onwards, every major suffrage bill brought before Parliament was defeated. This was chiefly because neither of the leading politicians of the day, William Gladstone and Benjamin Disraeli, cared to confront the implacable Queen Victoria's firm opposition to the women's movement. Despite the considerable support that existed, women were still denied the right to vote in any parliamentary elections.

Throughout many areas of the world, including Britain, women were legally the property of men. If not married, they were subservient to their eldest male relative and had no legal rights over their own property, their bodies or their lives. Repression, bodily mutilation, arranged marriages, and often forced marriages were considered acceptable practices. As property, females could be bought and sold into slavery or prostitution. Problematical wives were 'put away', incarcerated, or murdered. The founding of colleges for women, such as Girton, and the passing of the Married Women's Property Act were major steps in acknowledging the rights of women in Britain. However, without the responsibility and the right to vote, the majority of the adult population were powerless to affect issues within their own country and unable to influence even their own lives except through the good offices of any beneficent man.

The birth of Vladimir Ilyich Lenin in 1870 was one amongst the millions that went unremarked in the great Russian Empire. The violent upheavals of the Franco-Prussian struggles, mainly instigated by the German Chancellor Bismarck, resulted in the dethronement of the French Emperor, the siege of Paris in 1870 and the triumphant march of German troops through Paris in January 1871. A few months later, rebellious French citizens manned the barricades before their rebellion was violently put down. This Franco-Prussian war raised concerns about the conditions of the British Army, which badly needed reform, and soon the practice of purchasing commissions was abolished. From then on, promotion was earned on merit.

As horizons widened, tales of exploration, discovery and development beyond their small island thrilled the British public. In 1871, the meeting on the shores of Lake Tanganyika of the Scottish missionary and explorer David Livingstone with the English reporter Henry Stanley excited more European interest in the vast African continent. Livingstone's eldest son, Robert, who was to have joined his father in 1863, had never reached Africa, travelling instead to the United States where he had died in 1864, fighting for the North in the American Civil War. David Livingstone died in 1873 after a bout of fever. After burying his heart under a giant mapundu tree, his two faithful helpers carried his embalmed body for nine months across 1,600km of the African continent so that it could be taken back to England. The tale of their devotion touched the British nation and, in a great Victorian funeral, Livingstone was buried in Westminster Abbey on 18 April 1874.

With the passing of the Merchant Shipping Act in 1875, 'the sailor's friend', reformer William Plimsoll, finally succeeded in putting his life-saving mark – known as the Plimsoll line – on every ship. From then on, the Plimsoll line had to be visible above water level so that no ship could be dangerously overloaded by unscrupulous owners.

British agricultural workers went on strike for more wages, iron workers in south Wales struck in protest at a proposal to lower their wages and vast numbers of people emigrated to America and Canada in search of a better life in the New World. In 1878, William Booth renamed his mission organisation to create the Salvation Army, giving shelter and food to the needy and determinedly dealing with problems of prostitution and drunkenness.

In the year that Winston Churchill was born, Ethel's stepfather, 60-year-old George Storer, stood as a Conservative Party candidate in the 1874 general election and was elected, unopposed, as Member of Parliament for South Nottinghamshire. Ethel was then 17 and, as she later recorded, she had grown up in a political atmosphere and so naturally she read about debates in the House of Commons.

There were many changes and developments during George Storer's tenure as an MP. Refrigeration went into industrial production, eventually enabling frozen meat to be transported across the globe to Britain. An agricultural depression created unrest amongst labourers who were earning less than industrial workers. Reform of the law courts was under way and acts were passed to combat slum housing and also to codify sanitary laws.

In 1875, Ethel's older sister Clara, then aged 20, married 32-year-old Charles John Myers, of Dunningwell, eldest son of the Reverend Myers of Flintham and Fisketon. Charles was a military man. Having trained at Sandhurst, he had served as a Lieutenant of the 39th Foot regiment in 1866, stationed in Bermuda until 1869. He had retired just before the regiment was posted to India in 1870. Having property in Cumberland, Charles had then purchased a commission in the Royal Cumberland and Lincolnshire 34th Regiment. Following the death of his father that year, he had inherited responsibilities and property in Nottinghamshire and Lincolnshire, as well as the Dunningwell Estate in Cumbria.

Clara's marriage took place at Thoroton in the prettily decorated church, with eight bridesmaids in attendance. Paths were strewn with flowers and archways of flowers were erected by the villagers. The wedding breakfast was attended by sixty guests and the couple were presented with several numerous and costly gifts.

Following the wedding breakfast at Thoroton, the couple set off on honeymoon to Scotland and a few days later went to begin their married life at Dunningwell. They were greeted on the Green by tenantry and villagers who had erected a triumphal arch decorated with sheaves of wheat and symbolic agricultural emblems signifying the industry of the district. Horses were detached from the carriage and a presentation made by the Dunningwell tenants of a handsome Bible mounted in antique Morocco leather, and a silver mounted flagon by the Dunningwell servants. After appropriate speeches of gratitude from the groom, the carriage was then drawn by hand to the Dunningwell home. A few days later, a supper and ball were held in the Public Room on the Green for the tenantry and neighbours, with around 160 people attending the event. Dancing commenced at 8.00 pm and ended at 1.00 am.

The estate at Dunningwell included the old Queen Anne family holiday home house at the foot of a hill, known as Old Dunningwell. The new young bride, Clara, insisted on having a new 'modern' house built on top of a hill at Dunningwell and persuaded Charles to sell his Nottinghamshire estate. In its heyday, the property consisted of four acres of garden, fifteen acres of woodland, with five full time gardeners employed to care for the garden and grounds.

On 10 March 1876, Alexander Graham Bell uttered the words, 'Mr Watson, come here, I want you!' in the first electrical transmission of the human voice. The age of the telephone had begun; it was to change the world, as was the invention of the safety bicycle.

Russia pressed closer and the Afghanistan wars raged. Now owned by the British Empire, the Kimberley diamond mines in South Africa were proving productive. In 1876, Sir Henry Wickham collected rubber seeds from the wild trees of the Amazon jungles and had them planted in Kew Gardens. These emergent young trees were transferred to Ceylon and the Malay Peninsula, where they formed the base of the natural rubber plantation industry which was to affect so many aspects of British industry. The Ambulance Association, later to be known as the St John's Ambulance Brigade, was formed.

The opening of the Suez Canal proved vital for developing strong links with the East and all its riches and, by 1877, Queen Victoria was declared Empress of India and the British Empire had annexed the Transvaal. The Zulu wars began, and troubles were brewing in Ireland as nationalists aimed to reform the repressive Land Laws.

Ethel's school friends from her days at Middlethorpe school, the Wilkinsons, were by this time firmly associated with forward-thinking women such as the Garrett family. Despite opposition and difficulties, Fanny Wilkinson became Britain's first female landscape architect and her sister Louisa married into the Garrett family, becoming sister-in-law to Millicent and Elizabeth. The Garrett women were lively freethinkers and actively interested in politics. Millicent Garett had married the political reformer Henry Fawcett and became active in social reform and the women's suffrage movement. Elizabeth Garrett had married in 1871 to become Elizabeth Garrett Anderson and, with determination and perseverance, she had become Britain's first female doctor. It is highly probable that through her schooltime friendships Ethel Manson was exposed to the ideas, ideals, and influence of these exceptional and intelligent women reformers.

Unlike many of her contemporaries, Ethel Gordon Manson was not unduly concerned with finding a husband but was intent on a career outside the home. In 1878, by the time she was 21, she was determined to embark upon one of the few feasible careers available at the time to an educated woman – the developing field of nursing.

# Chapter 2

# Women, Work, Medicine, and Nursing up to the 1870s

While scientific discoveries and industrialisation rapidly advanced, social changes in Britain went at a slower pace. Many women began to protest at the unfairness of a system which awarded total legal rights over their lives and their bodies to men. In order to be heard and to have any serious influence within society, women needed to be able to vote. Without the power of the vote, they were impotent – unable to affect politics or social reform in any truly meaningful manner. In the nineteenth century, women began to demand the opportunities which nowadays are taken so much for granted. They wanted the opportunity to obtain education up to university level and to be able to work and earn enough to survive independently.

The significance of withholding the vote from over half the adult population was never fully appreciated by those who had always been able to take such a right for granted. In *The Social Position of Women in England 1885–1914: A Bibliography*, O. R. McGregor wrote:

> emancipation of women is one of the most striking aspects of the industrial phase of social development. Equally striking is its neglect in present-day writing. It has neither attracted comprehensive sociological analysis nor acquired status as an established theme of the history books.

Most historians completely neglected the role of women, with no insight to women's lives or any understanding of their powerlessness and consequent frustrations within society. It was not considered extraordinary when, in 1950, historian David Thompson published a book, *England in the Nineteenth Century*, which included only three references to women, writing merely that the major abuses in the employment of women and children had been removed. A brief mention of the fact that women got the vote in 1918 was followed by a short paragraph on women's suffrage, and a suggestion that 'the Great War saved this country from Ireland, the working classes and women'.

Industrialisation provided places for women workers in factories, giving them a degree of economic and social freedom. For the first time, many women received regular wages and were able to meet and interact with other women outside the home environment. However, by virtue of their supposed inferiority, women and children were paid far lower wages than men and as a consequence it became easier for them to find work. As well as the long working hours, these women endured poor housing, excessive childbearing, and the tragedy of a high infant death rate, but at least they could become independent wage-earners. The unmarried woman or the widow was no longer forced to rely on relatives for support or to apply for parish poor relief.

Lord Ashley, in a debate on the Factories Bill 1842, quoted from a letter:

> Mr. E., a manufacturer, informed me that he employs females exclusively at his power looms – it is so universally; he gives a decided preference to married females, especially those who have families at home dependent on them for support; they are attentive, docile more so than unmarried females, and are compelled to use their utmost efforts to procure the necessities of life.

Women formed the greater part of the night shift, not only because they were cheaper but believed to be 'more easily induced to undergo severe bodily fatigue than men'. Unsurprisingly, wages for men remained depressed as long as female labour was cheap. In the preface of *Women's Work*, Lady Dilke wrote in 1894: 'Colossal fortunes are built up in large measure by the enforced labour of women and children who are encouraged … in suicidal rivalry with their husbands and fathers in the labour market … Women have entered the labour scene as blacklegs.'

This preferential treatment had a detrimental effect on the menfolk who were discriminated against. They found difficulty in keeping their jobs after the age of 40 and Lord Ashley alludes to the number of 'ex-spinners reduced to hawking nuts, oranges and boiled sheep's feet or selling sand'.

Lord Ashley saw the factory situation in 1842 as causing a reversal in the natural family order:

> The females not only occupy the places of men; they are forming various clubs and associations, and gradually acquiring all those privileges which are held to be the proper position of the male sex. What is the ground on which the woman says she will pay no attention to her duties, nor give the obedience which is owing to her husband? Because on her devolves the labour that ought to fall to his share.

In spite of this thoughtless assumption that all women were married, throughout the nineteenth century and the first half of the twentieth century, women outnumbered men, particularly in the older age groups, mainly because the male death rate was higher than that of women – partly as a result of accidents and of wars. Another factor was the effect of emigration as a large number of working men went overseas to seek a better life. Eventually men began to organise themselves into workers' groups and began to implement change within their workplaces.

Josephine Butler, social reformer and promoter of women's education, had noted in 1866 that facts in society had changed faster than its conventions, with nearly a quarter of wives working outside their homes and with marriage being perceived as an exceedingly precarious means of subsistence. There were also 2.5 million widows and spinsters who needed to support themselves. She wrote:

> Two and a half million of Englishwomen without husbands, 'working for their own subsistence.' This is not an accident; it is a new order of things ... The desire for education, which is widely felt by English women, and which has begun to find its expression in practical ways is a desire which springs ... from the conviction that, for many women, to get knowledge is the only way to get bread.

Very few women continued professional work after marriage and in England, until the second half of the twentieth century, no hospital matron retained her post after marriage. Work was seen as a means of support for the unmarried woman and it was mainly the middle-class woman who began to demand education.

Only the most determined middle-class women were able to contemplate a career and the 25- year-old Florence Nightingale found her environment hostile when she unsuccessfully attempted to enter nursing at Salisbury. She wrote with frustration:

> Nothing will be done this year at all events, and I do not believe ever; and no advantage that I see comes of my living on, excepting that one becomes less and less of a young lady every year. O weary days, O evening that seem never to end! For how many years have I watched the drawing room clock and thought it would never reach ten!

Only when she was 31, and her family was convinced she would never marry, was she allowed to go to study nursing for three months in 1851. The Crimea and her deep involvement in that theatre of war came two years later.

Another determined woman was England's first woman doctor, Elizabeth Garrett Anderson, who suffered similar frustration to her ambitions and wrote later:

> I was a young girl living at home with nothing to do in what authors call 'comfortable circumstances'. But I was wicked enough not to be

comfortable. I was full of energy and vigour, and of the discontent which goes with unemployed activities. The obscure trouble of a baffled instinct as Coleridge finely calls it … Everything seemed wrong to me.

There were very few employment opportunities for an educated woman. While it was considered acceptable for women of labouring classes to work in factories or mines, middle-class women who aspired to support themselves with gainful employment were derided as unfeminine by men – and also by some other women.

Lady clerks were taken on by city companies such as the Prudential Insurance Society, city firms, stores, and railway companies. The supply of clerks exceeded demand and unscrupulous employers were able to offer increasingly lower salaries. The persistent and effective social reformer, Josephine Butler, noted when telegraph companies were first formed the pay of a female clerk was 8/- rising to 14/-. However, the throng of applicants was so great that this was lowered to 5/- and, when the government took over the telegraphs, the women clerks were dismissed because they did not have a vote to bestow on government candidates.

For some women, the only possible suitable employment was as a governess. In 1868, Josephine Butler noted that governesses were often offered a comfortable home, but no salary, and that one advertisement for a nursery governess on those conditions attracted 300 applicants. People were realising that only proper education could lead to emancipation and the only way for women to play a full role in the world was for them to have the right to vote. Gradually the call for female suffrage grew louder.

The Reform Bill of 1832 had confined votes to qualifying 'male persons'. Protesters laid a petition before Parliament asking that, with the necessary property qualification, every unmarried woman should be allowed to vote. Women found a parliamentary champion in John Stuart Mill in 1866 and in the early days the women's suffrage movement was sustained by a relatively small group of educated women. These included

Emily Davies and doctor Elizabeth Garrett Anderson, who delivered the petition for female suffrage to John Stuart Mill at the House of Commons. Florence Nightingale did not sign this petition, although, much later, she did eventually subscribe to women's suffrage.

Queen Victoria did not approve. Secure from the realities of middle-class life, she committed her opinions on the subject in writing:

> The Queen is most anxious to enlist everyone who can speak or write or join in checking the mad wicked folly of 'Women's Rights', with all its attendant horrors, on which her poor feeble sex is bent, forgetting every sense of womanly feeling and propriety.

Eventually, in 1869, women taxpayers were granted the right to vote in municipal elections, and in the following years women became eligible to sit on county and city councils. However, the right to vote in parliamentary elections was still denied to women, in spite of the considerable and increasing support for their cause. With the exception of 1874, a bill for female suffrage was laid before Parliament every year in the 1870s. As the subject began to be taken more seriously, so the objections to it grew. Initially the petition was hampered by the lack of educated women able to organise a political movement. Support gradually grew from both political parties for the bill, but submission of a Private Member's Bill was complicated and difficult.

Women were making inroads into medicine, but the fight for respect and acceptance from colleges and patients was long and hard. A Medical Register instituted by Act of Parliament in 1858 provided for registration of all doctors who were in practice at that time. Elizabeth Blackwell had graduated in medicine in New York State in 1849, before opening a dispensary for immigrant women and children in New York. When the 1858 Act was passed, she returned to England to have her name put on the British Register.

The example of Elizabeth Blackwell inspired Elizabeth Garrett to become the first woman doctor to take her training in this country. When asked, 'Why not be a nurse?' she replied, 'I prefer to earn a thousand rather than twenty pounds a year.' Elizabeth Garrett began her career at the Middlesex Hospital, initially as a lady probationer nurse. In spite of much determined effort, she failed to get permission to graduate from either London or St Andrews University. It is interesting to note that she experienced no difficulty in getting private tuition – discouraged from earning money, there was no prohibition on her spending it! Undaunted, she found a loophole to enable her to achieve her ambition of practising medicine in Britain. In 1815, a royal charter had been granted to the Society of Apothecaries, giving them the right to examine and license 'all persons desiring to practice medicine'. Taking advantage of this, Elizabeth become licensed in 1865. Swift action was taken afterwards by the Society to close this loophole. The comment by Charles Newman illustrates the attitude of the time:

> it was thought natural, in a way, for women to nurse; they had always done it in the home; but for the theoretically subordinate sex to assume the function of making decisions in a Victorian world was quite another matter.

Among the early group of women who emerged to promote women's suffrage, the names of Emily Davis, Elizabeth Garrett Anderson, and Barbara Bodichon are prominent. Emily Davies was an educational reformer and eventually became Mistress of Girton College for women in Cambridge, which had been founded in 1869. She was a close friend of the first English woman doctor, Elizabeth Garrett Anderson, and both of them worked tirelessly to persuade and promote women into the fields of education and medicine.

Louisa, sister of Fanny Wilkinson (the first female landscape architect), married into the Garrett family. Both sisters had been schooled at Middlethorpe and it is highly likely that Ethel Manson was influenced by these school friends as well as their kindly father, respected physician Dr Matthew Wilkinson. Elizabeth Garrett Anderson's younger sister,

Millicent, married Henry Fawcett, political economist and reformer. Henry Fawcett had been blinded in an accident in 1858, became a professor at Cambridge, a Liberal MP, Postmaster General from 1880 and played a great part in campaigning for women's suffrage. Barbara Bodichon, the multi-talented daughter of radical MP Leigh Smith, was another one of their friends, and she studied at Bedford College London, before becoming one of the founders of Girton College.

Another reformer in this circle and also one of Elizabeth Garret Anderson's patients was Josephine Gray. She married George Butler, the Canon of Winchester, and as well as promoting women's education, as Josephine Butler she relentlessly crusaded against licensed brothels and white-slave traffic. She also fought a long and eventually successful campaign against the Contagious Diseases Act. This iniquitous Act made every woman in seaports and military towns liable for compulsory examination for venereal disease. Discussions on the merits of the Act were long and heated between politicians in Parliament.

Surprisingly, in 1873, Elizabeth Garrett Anderson did not think the time was right for women to obtain their medical education in England. In a letter to *The Times*, she recommended they undertook a course in Paris, where she had obtained her degree. Having just endured, with six other women, four years of hard work, humiliation, riot, lawsuit, and eventual failure in her examination, aspirant doctor Sophia Jex-Blake responded with outrage.

Sophia Jex-Blake was sister to the headmaster of Rugby school and had become a tutor of mathematics at Queens College for Women London before studying medicine in New York under Elizabeth Blackwell. She fought her way into Edinburgh University and was allowed to matriculate in 1869 along with five of her female Edinburgh colleagues. However, the university authorities reversed their decision in 1873.

Determined, Sophia obtained her medical qualifications in Dublin and opened the London School of Medicine for Women in 1874. In 1876, an Act was passed enabling medical corporations to license women. In 1886, Sophia founded a medical school in Edinburgh and from 1894 women were allowed to graduate from there into medicine. It was 1883 before London University awarded a medical degree to women and, unsurprisingly following all the difficulties, by 1894 only 100 women were qualified in medicine. In view of the prejudices against them, and the conditions within medicine at the time, it is remarkable that women were able to gain admission to the Register when they did. The mighty Stock Exchange managed to hold out against women until the mid-twentieth century.

In the first half of the nineteenth century, those patients who could afford it were treated at home and nursed by their families. The poor and the destitute sick were cared for in hospitals. Anaesthetics were unknown before the 1840s; bacteriology as a science did not exist until well into the second half of the century. No change in nursing was possible until the development and major improvements in medicine and surgery.

The physician was the educated man who practiced internal medicine, chiefly by consultation and prescription. When the writer Emily Brontë was dying of tuberculosis, her sister Charlotte wrote to a London specialist who gave advice and prescriptions without even seeing the patient. Surgeons were supposed to only practice external medicine. Until 1812, the Royal College of Physicians required a mere six months of work in hospital, and the student chose his own lecturers and work, 'walking the wards' in search of knowledge. Until the Medical Register was established in 1859, the public found it difficult to distinguish between trained and untrained doctors.

A correspondent in *The Spectator* in 1969 wrote: 'medicine in the shape of actually doing anything to cure patients is the invention of the past hundred years. Before this the account is mainly a melancholy history of cruelty, superstition and ignorance.'

The nurse had been considered no more than a domestic servant but, by encouraging educated women to enter hospital work, Florence Nightingale founded a workforce of dedicated nurses. She inspired women to follow her example and did much to highlight the many challenges to be faced. Nursing was at last becoming organised and governments were able to base their health policies on hospitals and sick beds.

In 1902, the journal of the League of Saint Bartholomew's Hospital published the following account from a member of their first school of nursing, in 1877 which reveals hospital life of that time and is worth quoting at length:

> You want to hear something about my training? Well, I came in on May 1st 1877, just five and twenty years ago. I was one of a batch of twelve probationers, the first to be trained in St. Bartholomew's Hospital. Before we came, there was no sort of training for the nurses, and of nursing as you understand it now there was simply none. The Matron, Mrs. Drake, greatly disapproved of such innovations as 'lady-nurses', and tried hard to dissuade me from entering when I came up to be interviewed. There was no entrance examination. We all arrived one morning and put on our uniform. What was it? The present probationer's uniform, with the exception of the cap, which were small caps without strings. This was quite different from the uniform of the so-called 'staff-nurses', who wore brown merino dresses, aprons without bibs, collars, no cuffs, caps or no caps as they liked, and when worn, of any description. I remember hearing some weeks after we arrived that the head-dispenser had pronounced us 'an ornament to the square.' That night I was sent to Harley where I shared a room opening into the ward (the dressing room) with the staff nurse. I did not get much rest. To begin with my room-mate was very drunk and very sick. Being ignorant of the symptoms, I wasted much pity on her. When I did fall off to sleep, I was wakened by frightful screams and shouts of 'Murder' 'Fire' I proceeded to wake up my companion, who growled 'Be quiet. It's only 178'.

Drunkenness was very common amongst the staff-nurses who were chiefly women of the 'charwoman' type, frequently of bad character with little or no education, and few of them with even an elementary knowledge of nursing. Some of them might have worked previously at some other hospital but, as often as not, they had no experience whatever when engaged as 'staff nurses'. One woman, I remember, who came some little time after I did and under whom I worked, had been a lady's maid, and had never done a day's nursing. She was, however, of a decidedly superior class to any of the others, and was, moreover, quite respectable. It was very usual for the friends to bring in presents of gin to bribe the nurses to be kind to the patients. The worst women we had were those who used to come in to look after very bad cases, more particularly at night. They were called 'night extras'. They were mostly dreadful persons, possessing neither character nor ability, who used to apply here for work much as women now apply for charring.

Among the Sisters, there was already some improvement. Some there were still of whose virtues the less said the better, and some were wholly untrained – a knowledge of nursing not being in those days a necessary qualification for that special work. Sister Eyes was the ophthalmic Sister – the first to be appointed for that special work. A few also had been trained at the 'Nightingale' Home. We should not think much now of the training they had had, but it was a good deal for the time. They also had had considerable experience, and were, moreover, clever and capable women of superior character. Chief among them was Sister Matthew (Miss Witton), better known now as 'Old Sister Faith', and with her I must mention Sisters Elizabeth Colston and Sitwell (afterwards 'Henry'). Of 'Old Sister Faith' many stories are still told. She was a great character and a keen and capable nurse. She took a great interest in her nurses, and taught them all she could, if they wished to learn. Many years later than the time of which I am speaking, when asked one day if the nurses were still addicted to drink, she replied – 'No, nowadays it's not drinking – it's flirting.' Then, it must be remembered that, among the sisters who had no training at all, there were several very good women, whose long experience in the wards had rendered them fairly capable nurses. The first night superintendents were appointed also at the time our training began, in the persons of Miss Sleigh (now Sister President) and Miss Irving (afterwards for a short time Sister of Hope Ward). One or two of the other Sisters had been 'Sisters' (otherwise wardresses) at Newgate Gaol. What did they wear? Blue merino dresses, without either caps or aprons. I was the first sister who always wore both, and, indeed for some years I always removed my apron before going to dinner.

How were we taught? Well, by the Sisters – very little. (The staff-nurses were not capable of teaching us anything). Few of the Sisters both could and would teach us. Sir Dyce Duckworth or Mr. Willett lectured to us or gave us a practical demonstration once a week. Mr. Willett used to have his out-patient children and teach us to bandage, to put on splints, to make and apply plasters, bandages and so on. Sir Dyce would take us into the wards and give us a lesson on bed-making, poultice-making or on the contents of the doctor's cupboard, or down to the bathrooms where he and old Williams, the bath-man, used to show us the best way to get the patients in and out of the bath, and how to prepare special baths of various kinds. We were known as 'Ducky's lambs'. The present bathrooms off the wards were only just being built. Before we had them, all patients who were in fit condition in the wards were bathed in the baths under the out-patient department. The only baths in the wards were in the kitchens, and were covered with wooden covers which often served as a table on which to carve the dinners.

Then we picked up what we could, and the resident staff and students taught us a good deal. You see, we were quite a novelty, and everyone took a great interest in us. Dr. Griffith I think, taught me to take temperatures. He was a dresser. The thermometers in use then were very much larger than those we use now, and had to be read while in position, as they ran down at once when removed from the mouth or armpit. They cost 12/6 each. The Sisters and nurses never used a thermometer; the dressers and clerks took the temperatures when required. We probationers were expected to learn the use of clinical thermometers, but there was generally a row if Sister caught us with one.

How did we get on with the staff-nurses? On the whole – very well. You see our coming brought about several improvements. To begin with, before then, all the three nurses (night and day) shared the one small bedroom, sharing 'Box and Cox'. When we came, the 'night home' was arranged to accommodate the night nurses, which left only the two day nurses to sleep in the ward bedroom. Then a dining room was also made (part of our present library), where breakfast and dinner were provided. Tea we had in the ward (not in the kitchen), and for supper we had only what we chose to get for ourselves before going to bed. Before we came, all the nurses' food was cooked and eaten in the ward, as also the Sisters'. No, the Sisters had no dinner provided. They were given a chop (uncooked) on Sundays only. They lived entirely in their rooms, which were half the size most of them are now.

What hours? We were on duty from 7a.m. until 10pm. Twice a week we were supposed to go off duty for two hours, 6 to 8pm, and to have half a day (3pm – 9pm) once a fortnight. I say supposed, as we never got off punctually; the work could not be finished in time. When we came in we went on duty again until 10 'o' clock.

How does the work now compare with the work then? Well, of course, nursing, as you understand it now, was utterly unknown. Patients were not nursed then, they were 'attended to' more or less; but there was only one nurse in each side of the ward and the work was very hard – lockers, locker-boards, and tables, of course, to scrub every day. No, we did not, as a rule, scrub floors though I have scrubbed the whole of the front-ward of Matthew (Faith) on a special occasion before 6am. Luke was the only ward where the floor was scrubbed daily, each nurse doing her half, and Sister herself lending a hand if they were very busy. (Luke was considered a particularly smart ward in those days, and Sister always wore a black silk dress when she went round with the Visiting Physician). The patients had their beds made once a day, the bad cases had their sheets drawn at night. In Matthew all the patients got out of bed every day, even the 'typhoids' – it was considered rather smart. Then you thought nothing of having fourteen or fifteen poultices to change. All wounds, of course, suppurated, and required dressing or poulticing twice or three times a day. I well remember Mr. Willet saying when lecturing us on wounds 'There are three modes of healing; the first, most to be desired, but never seen, by first intention; the second, by granulation and the third, which is always seen, by suppuration.'

We had breakfast and dinner in the home; otherwise, when off duty, if we did not go out, we sat in the ward kitchens or our bedrooms. The food was fairly good. There was no one to overlook our behaviour or to see that we went to bed at the right time or anything of that sort. Indeed, I often sat up very late, and when in Faith, went round frequently with the Sister and the H.P. when they made the night round. I learnt a good deal then. I generally had to write my lectures out before I got up in the morning between five and six. It was the only quiet time and the only time of the day when my head was clear enough; at night I was too tired.

At the end of the year we passed an examination held much on the same lines as now, but I believe marks were not awarded by the Matron until after Miss Manson came. We were awarded certificates and offered posts as staff nurses, which few were bold enough to accept on account of the existing conditions of things.

We objected to associating constantly and sharing rooms with the staff nurses, to changing our clean cotton uniform for their brown staff-dresses, and to carrying soiled linen from the wards to the laundry (which the staff-nurses then had to do), and various other things. The Treasurer promised to try and alter these things, and did so by degrees. One or two out of every batch of probationers (they came in every three months) stayed on after passing the examination. Then Miss Machin, who became Matron in 1879, increased the period of training to two years, so that we had a certain number of second-year nurses on whom we could depend. It was not, however, until Miss Manson came in 1881 that the old, untrained Sisters and nurses were gradually weeded out and the training lengthened to three years. A tremendous change? Yes, greater than you can imagine. I have really no words in which to describe the state the Hospital was in when I came as a probationer, and, if I had, you would say the account was not fit for publication. It was many years before the nursing staff was treated with anything approaching respect.

Such a valuable first-hand account reveals the remarkable tenacity and devotion to their work shown by these pioneer nurses. Undaunted by the prospect of hard work, this was the world that Ethel wished to enter and which she helped change for the better.

# Chapter 3

# Old Medicine, the New Nurse, and Promotion: 1878–1897

The final forty years of the nineteenth century had seen annexation of vast areas of land in Africa, the Far East, and the Pacific. The British Raj governed India and the Britons who ventured into that massive continent to make their fortunes suffered badly from the exacting climate. While trying valiantly to maintain their own traditions in this foreign environment, they fell prey to horrendous diseases of which they had little understanding. Newspapers were full of helpful but totally useless advice with advertisements extolling the efficacy of wearing garments such as the 'cholera belt'. It is a testament to Victorian tenacity that any one of the British abroad survived to achieve anything.

In the early nineteenth century, efforts were still being made to find an all-embracing medical theory, and doctors strove to find a single system to account for disease. Lack of cadavers for student teaching meant anatomy was imperfectly understood. Experimentation and observation were discouraged and a rigid caste system separated physicians, surgeons and apothecaries.

The physician practiced internal medicine and earned his fee by consultation and prescribing, gaining his knowledge in the library rather than at the bedside. The chief assets required by a surgeon were boldness and physical strength in pre-anaesthetic days, and operations were restricted to what a conscious patient could bear and to the speed of the surgeon. The apothecary was the druggist who made up the medicines ordered by the physicians and he often prescribed the medication himself. The amount of medical knowledge was minute;

philosophy and botany were important subjects and some drugs were added to the Pharmacopoeia simply by virtue of having been used as remedies by village wise-women.

The Diploma of the College of Surgeons was given without any clinical test, and no examination in medicine or *materia medica*. The licentiateship of the Apothecaries Company did not imply any knowledge of anatomy or surgery. The granting of titles provided a lucrative source of income and, understandably, examining bodies were easily satisfied. Eighteen independent and uncontrolled licensing authorities all competed with one another for candidates and fees, and consequently standards were often deplorably low. The surgeon was almost entirely concerned with external conditions, not diagnosis, and the commonest operation was that of amputation for trauma or malignancy. Bleeding was considered essential for health and it was a usual occurrence for country folk to come into market, get bled in the doctor's surgery until they fainted and then, recovering, drive the horse and cart home again.

In 1846, Robert Liston at University College Hospital, London, was the first to use ether as an anaesthetic when performing a leg amputation. In 1847, in Edinburgh, Sir James Simpson began to use chloroform on his patients. The first British professional anaesthetist was John Snow – the doctor famous for his work on mapping cases of cholera and his ordering the removal of the handle of Broad Street water pump, which stopped a cholera epidemic of 1854. Official royal sanction was given to anaesthetics by Queen Victoria when she accepted chloroform administered by John Snow during the birth of her eighth child, Prince Leopold, in 1853.

Florence Nightingale had been recognised as a heroine and a nursing pioneer following her work, when in her thirties, in the Crimea War (1853–1856). However, she was not the first to undertake the task of nursing wounded soldiers. There had been a long history of women, mostly soldiers' wives, accompanying military campaigns throughout the ages. In the British Army, women were not encouraged on campaigns but some wives were listed as unpaid camp followers. Desperate to help their menfolk, some managed to find employment as regimental cooks and laundresses as well as untrained nurses. George Washington had mustered untrained nurses to work in the American Civil War, their wages being $2 a month and, in 1776, the ideal ratio being ten patients to each nurse.

A mixed-race daughter of a Scottish soldier, the remarkable Mary Seacole (1805–1881), from Jamaica, offered her nursing experience to Florence Nightingale but was firmly rebuffed. Undeterred, she made her way to the Crimea, arriving in 1855 at Balaklava, where she opened a hotel housing a good clean canteen for the troops. Being independent, she had the freedom to travel to the battle front with her two mules, carrying medications and food. She was able to bring comfort and medicine to the injured and dying and food to men who had been fighting and fasting for hours. By the end of the war, she was left bankrupt, but her remarkable work had been recorded by journalists at the front and an appeal was raised to help refund her losses in the Crimea. Her work was acknowledged by Queen Victoria and a fund was set up to ensure she could survive in relative comfort until her death in London in 1881.

In the 1850s, the mortality rate for the removal of an ovarian cyst was over 30 per cent and the death rate following amputation in military hospitals was between 75 per cent and 90 per cent In the early nineteenth century, the general public were unable to distinguish between the trained and the untrained doctor because any person, licensed or not, could practise in England and Wales. This horrifyingly unsafe practice changed with the publication of the Medical Register in 1859. However, entry to the register did not require more than a superficial knowledge of medical matters. When the pioneer British woman doctor Elizabeth Garrett took her MD in Paris in 1870, she was questioned not only on treatment of pneumonia and the management of extra-uterine pregnancy, but on taking of footprints in police cases, the preparation of arsenical compounds, and the classification of fishes!

Until the second half of the nineteenth century, there was no understanding of the causes of the wound infections which invariably occurred and which were thought to be a normal part of the healing process. Although bacteria were seen under the microscope, they were not understood to be the specific cause of disease. The cause of sepsis was unknown and some doctors thought the disease process produced bacteria and believed that bad smells, exhalations from drains and sewers and other bad air, produced diseases. Sometimes, coincidentally, getting rid of the cause of smells did work because the clearing of cesspits and stagnant water removed the carrier mechanism of disease.

The theory of 'laudable pus' was firmly believed, some discharges perceived to be better than others. It was observed that the frank pus of infection by staphylococcus, such as occurs in boils, was better than the thin musty discharge of gas gangrene that led inevitably to death. Meanwhile, for hundreds of years in Africa it had been well understood that unseen 'small things' caused disease as well as causing the fermentation of cheese and beer. Eventually, in the western world, Louis Pasteur was able to show that putrefaction was due to bacteria and strove to destroy them by antiseptic dressings.

Ignaz Semmelweis, a Hungarian obstetrician, had demonstrated that hand washing made a marked decrease in the death rate of patients. Sadly, his superiors did not agree and resented being told that they were directly responsible for the high death rate. He was forced to retire from Vienna to Budapest where, ironically, he contracted fatal septicaemia. His work was not wasted, however, as the English surgeon Joseph Lister heard of his achievements and in 1865 began soaking surgical dressings in carbolic acid (phenol) and also used it to clean his hands and his instruments. Not until he was able to prove consistent and repeated success with his new antisepsis techniques did other surgeons begin to use Lister's methods.

At this time, drunkenness was common among the staff nurses in hospitals, who were generally ill-educated with barely an elementary knowledge of nursing. Until 1877, there was little difference between a nurse and a domestic servant. Patients were simply attended to, ward furniture was scrubbed and cleaned, beds changed daily, and numerous sodden poultices were changed frequently.

The practice of medicine was undergoing enormous developments and these changes had a direct effect on the requirements within nursing. The metamorphosis from sick attendant to professional nurse took place in last quarter of the nineteenth century. As result of Florence Nightingale's impressive work in the Crimea, a testimonial fund had been established but, declining to accept a personal gift, she agreed that the money raised should be used to establish a school for nurse training where her beliefs and ideas on nursing could be put into practice. St Thomas's Hospital was selected and there, in 1860, the first nursing school in England was established.

In 1878, when she was 21, Ethel Manson was too young to be accepted by a general hospital, so she began her training, from April to September, as a paying Probationer at the Children's Hospital, Nottingham. Ethel's own lively description of her interview with the matron gives an insight into her persuasive character.

> I presented an offering of great odorous Czar violets – fresh from the home garden – she buried her face in them with delight. A few words sufficed to express the imperative desire for work on my part, and the instinctive appreciation of my needs on the part of the matron. I offered ten stone of perfect physical development, youth, and boundless enthusiasm, and in spite of appearances (low be it spoken, I had made my call in very short kilted skirts, Norfolk jacket, billycock hat, and very neat boots, and to these incongruities may be added a buttonhole, a stick, and a 'waist'!) She thought the offer sound, and we struck a bargain then and there.

Nottingham Children's Hospital had been founded in 1869 and there was a family connection for Ethel with Nottingham General Hospital. Dr John Storer, well respected grandfather of her stepfather George Storer, and the first President of the Bromley House Library, had been an influential medical practitioner in Nottingham. Nearly a century earlier, in 1781, he had taken a leading role in the founding of Nottingham General Hospital. In 1878, Ethel's mother Harriette and George Storer attended a ball in Nottingham devised to raise funds for the Nottingham Children's Hospital where Ethel was a probationary nurse.

Poor living conditions in the town at that time contributed to a high mortality rate amongst children, due to consumption (pulmonary tuberculosis), measles, whooping cough, scarlet fever, diarrhoea, and typhus. The life expectancy for a child in the slum areas of the town was fourteen years and a hospital for the children of the poor was desperately required. Before a child could be admitted, a parent was required to sign a humiliating declaration of poverty which had to be countersigned by a clergyman of their parish, or other minister of religion. Others who were not classified as poor had to pay for their nursing and treatment. Nursing was the responsibility of the Sisters of John's House until 1874 when they withdrew and a Lady Matron, a Miss Townsend, was appointed to manage the hospital.

The Children's Hospital was small, with two wards, one for boys and one for girls, of twelve cots each. Ethel enjoyed the work and described the Matron, Miss Minks, as 'the strictest disciplinarian and most able administrator' she had ever met. Miss Minks was evidently just as impressed with her new trainee and Ethel was allowed to deputise during the matron's holiday, doubtless finding the duties similar to the familiar ones of running a large household. In 1879, the Children's Hospital was one of the first buildings in Nottingham to be equipped with a telephone – a great improvement when it was necessary to contact doctors based at the General Hospital.

Later that year, Ethel continued her training as a paying probationer, which cost her £6.10. 0d for the year, at the Manchester Royal Infirmary. One of the eminent physicians at this Infirmary was Dr Mathew Wilkinson, although he died that year, in 1878. Dr Wilkinson had been the owner of Middlethorpe Hall School where Ethel had been educated and where she would have met Fanny Wilkinson, his daughter, who had family connections with the innovative and social reforming Garett family.

Meanwhile, in 1879, Ethel's stepfather, George Storer MP, spoke in detail in Parliament against the resolution to give the vote to women. He stated that 'ladies are perfectly satisfied with the domestic sphere in which they find themselves and in which many of them are such bright examples'. He did, however, note that they had 'science, art and literature – in which many of them excel so greatly, they have the hospital, they have district visiting'. He further suggested that women had no place in the 'dusty and soiled arena of political warfare'.

Conditions at Manchester Royal Infirmary were bleak and the work was demanding. Trainees were up at 6.00 am, scrubbing floors for two hours before beginning the work of the day. Records show that, in 1880, out of the fifty nurses engaged at Manchester, only fifteen made good, twenty were dismissed, six died, two failed in health, one left to be married, three left to 'better themselves', and three resigned. Many of those dismissed left because, as the record states bluntly, their 'health failed'. It took a strong constitution to withstand the rigours of hospital nursing.

Once again, Ethel was considered able and trustworthy enough to act up and take charge of the nearby Barnes Convalescent Home during the absence of the Matron. Testimonials from the Infirmary refer to her energy, tact in dealing with staff, and kindness to patients. A year later, at the end of her training and following a recommendation by Miss Minks, Ethel received a letter from Miss Swift, the Matron of the London Hospital, offering her the post of senior sister of the women's medical ward. Armed with an impressive bunch of testimonials, she went to London.

Ethel started at Whitechapel, London, in the middle of September 1879, as Sister of Charlotte Ward. The ward consisted of fifty-two beds, staffed by four nurses during the day and two at night, with one 'scrubber'. She lived in two rooms, a bedroom and sitting room adjoining the ward, and, as the ward sister, she was never off duty. Ward work was very physically demanding and included two daily ward rounds by the five house physicians. Ethel enjoyed the work and she got on well with medical staff. She would proudly recall that, whenever the hospital Committee toured the wards, they complimented her on the apple-pie order of her cupboards and on the freshness of the lovely flowers in her care. Her patients were noted to be happy, well nursed, and contented.

In December 1879, the collapse of the Tay Bridge, which resulted in over ninety train passengers being drowned, shocked the nation. In 1880, in order to standardise time throughout the country, Parliament ordered that all clocks be set at Greenwich Mean Time. The Employers' Liability Act enabled workers to obtain compensation for injuries which were not their own fault. The first telephone directory was published, containing 255 entries and electric tramcars arrived in London. The great innovator Marie Stopes was born in Edinburgh in 1880. Thomas Edison and his research team were busy developing electric light bulbs and electricity supply systems.

There were changes at the London Hospital when pretty 26-year-old Eva Luckes was appointed Matron in 1880. Educated at Malvern, Cheltenham College, and Dresden, Eva had not allowed a physical disablement to deter her ambitions for nursing. Work as a probationer at the Middlesex Hospital had proved too strenuous but, after a rest, she managed to complete training at the Westminster Hospital by 1878. She then gained short spells of experience at the London Hospital, Manchester Hospital for Sick Children, and Great Ormond Street Hospital for Sick Children before obtaining the post of Matron at the London Hospital. A sub-committee had already been formed to review the system and Eva set about reforming the standards of nursing. She sought advice from Florence Nightingale, whose cousin General Sir Lothian Nicolson was a governor of the hospital.

With Matron Luckes as her superior, Ethel Gordon Manson was Sister of Charlotte Ward at the London Hospital, and it was here that she met Dr Bedford Fenwick. He was a tall, handsome, and imposing man, inspiring many a female heart to flutter, including those of the new Matron Eva Luckes and of Ethel Manson.

The politician Disraeli died in 1881 – the same year that saw the abolition of flogging in the Army and Navy and the invention of a rolling machine to make cigarettes. The following year, the first public power station employing an electric generator was opened in London and a second such station was opened in New York City. Both unfortunately used systems which proved inefficient for long-distance electricity transmissions – but it was a start and proved the saying, 'anything man can imagine, man can achieve'. The British Parliament was illuminated with the new electric light in 1881 using technology developed by Joseph Swan. Eventually Swan and Edison formed a joint company and worked together on improving the distribution of electricity.

Back in the city slums of Britain, poverty reigned, and the accompanying diseases caused as a result of a lack of public health and hygiene standards were rife. In 1881, more than 100 people died of starvation in London. The working classes were enjoying the new pastime of attending football matches and the newly opened annual Blackpool illuminations, while the game of cricket was becoming more popular, but nothing could rival the national preoccupation with horse racing.

As well as the discoveries being made in the field of anaesthesia and in the prevention of infection, there were advances in protective community medicine. The first formal international health conference had been held in Paris in 1851 and was followed by a series of similar conferences aimed at drafting international quarantine regulations.

Confident and ambitious, eleven months after beginning her work at Whitechapel, Ethel applied for post of Matron at Richmond hospital but was unsuccessful. Undeterred by this setback in her career plans, she continued to look for a post as Matron. When, in 1881 she read an advert for a new Matron in the evening paper, she set off to put in her application in person the next morning. The excellent references from the London Hospital attesting to her intelligence and excellent managerial skills, combined with her persuasiveness and attractive appearance, ensured her immediate appointment. At 24 years of age, Ethel Gordon Manson was appointed Matron of St Bartholomew's Hospital, London, one of the largest and most famous voluntary hospitals in the country.

Before Ethel had returned from her interview, her Whitechapel colleagues had heard the good news of her prestigious appointment. The Chairman of the London Hospital welcomed her with a triumphant return by having a carriage and pair awaiting her when she alighted from the tram and her colleagues showered her with congratulations. In securing a most impressive post at one of London's main hospitals, Ethel certainly had achieved a major triumph and, despite her youth, was soon to prove herself worthy of such a great responsibility.

An article appeared in the London Hospital bulletin:

Miss Manson, for some one 'Sister Charlotte' at this hospital – has been appointed to a post of matron at St. Bartholomew's. The authorities at the latter hospital are very much to be congratulated on their selection, and the London loses a lady whose nursing ability and efficiency are excelled only by her kindness and urbanity. Upon hearing of this appointment, a spontaneous, though necessarily hurried movement was set on foot by those house-physicians and students who have been most intimately associated with Sister Charlotte in hospital work, to present her with some tangible though inadequate proof not only of their good wishes for her future happiness and success, but as an expression of the high opinion that they entertain for her in her official capacity, their esteem of her bright and charming personal character, and lastly, but not least, as a memento of her too short sojourn at the London. The present consisted of a drawing-room table, with china tea-service and all necessaries for afternoon tea.

St Bartholomew's had a long history of ministering to the sick. The hospital had been founded in 1123 by an English churchman of Frankish descent, Rahere, who had suffered and been cured of an attack of malarial fever while on pilgrimage to Rome. During his convalescence, he vowed to build a hospital and, on his return to London, he was granted a site at Smithfield by King Henry I. Rahere remained in charge of the hospital until he retired to a priory in 1137. A second Royal Charter was granted to the hospital by Henry VIII in 1546.

St Bartholomew's Hospital had witnessed many of the great and also the gorier moments of London history. In 1196, the Smithfield martyrs were burnt to death just outside its walls and there, in 1305, William Wallace was hanged, disembowelled and beheaded. In its shadow, Wat Tyler, the leader of the Peasants' Revolt against an unpopular poll tax, was killed in 1381, and Joan of Kent was burnt at the stake in 1550. 'Barts' was visited by the Plague in 1665 and only just managed to escape the worst of the Great Fire of London in 1666.

Nowadays the name 'Sister' is the only reminder of the former religious status of the hospital, and records show that in 1554 the sisters began to wear a distinctive blue livery. Winfred Hector, formerly Principal Tutor at 'Barts', gave a valuable history of the hospital in an article in 1973 in which she described the life of the hospital throughout the ages. With her permission, much of the following information is extracted from her article.

> When the Hospital was founded, there were eight brothers and four sisters living and working in the Hospital. They kept the rule of St. Augustine of Hippo, observed canonical requirements, and cared for the sick and the destitute, travelers and foundlings. Regular records started in 1549 and contain frequent mention of the sisters, which all helps to build up a picture of their work and life in the sixteenth century. It would appear that very few patients were dependent and totally confined to bed – mainly because medical knowledge was so primitive that most such helpless people died. The sisters kept their title but, after the second foundation, were lay women. A matron was in charge of eleven sisters, and

of the admission of patients to the wards. The first Matron was Rose Fisher who remained in the post until 1559. Her sisters wore blue, and one reference is to Matron's winter gown of red wool. The sisters worked on until old age stopped them, although it is recorded that one who retired because of infirmity in 1550 'received a benevolence of 8/4d'. Matron was concerned with the welfare of her nurses as well as that of her patients. Not all patients were housed on the premises; pregnant women were sent to a lying-in ward St. Thomas' Hospital, and other patients went to leper hospitals within the City.

It was the sister's responsibility to fetch the patient's food and drink from the buttery, to serve it to them and to feed the helpless. She also had the task of carrying the water until 1553. The ward sisters spun flax into yarn for the weavers to make into bed linen and up until 1678, Matron bought the hemp for spinning.

Rushes were strewn on the ward floors, and the patients slept on pallets filled with straw. Rushes and straw had to be burnt in the garden when soiled, and to control the smoke it was necessary to build a chimney in 1554. Until the middle of the seventeenth century the sisters washed all the patients' personal and bed linen. For this task they used wood ash up to 1687, when the Governors were then asked to permit the use of soap because wood ash had become very expensive. Available from whaling, soap had become cheaper, but it was a primitive product containing sand and soapwort.

The seventeenth century was an eventful time for London and the Hospital. The Civil War had little effect on the life of St. Bartholomew's; but when the Plague arrived in 1665 the two physicians took fright and left. The Matron, Margaret Blague, remained at her post, 'cooking soup and making comforts for her sick and poor'. By now nurses, or 'helpers' had appeared to lighten the sisters' work load.

The Great Fire came to the gates of the Hospital in 1666, destroying its properties. The consequent loss of revenue caused the hospital severe financial problems necessitating the closure of five of the fifteen wards and the discharge of their sisters. Things improved eventually and at the beginning of the eighteenth century a newly designed building arose. An illustration of Rahere Ward in 1832 shows the bedsteads were of wood. A contractor was required to keep the wards free of bugs; the floors were cleaned with brooms and sand. The mattresses and bolsters were stuffed with flock and round each bed were curtains of blue or yellow check lindsey. Wheelchairs, footstools and warming pans were in the ward which was lit by candlelight. It was a great luxury to have water pumped to each floor. Plunge baths were available, and patients were also taken to the Public Bath in Newgate Street.

By then the patients' daily diet consisted of twelve ounces of bread, eight ounces of beef or mutton, or butter and cheese, and three pints of beer which was still brewed in the Hospital. In addition, there was a pint of meat broth or porridge, with ale daily. The sisters compensated in part for dietetic deficiency by brewing a 'scurvy drink'. Flax spinning was a thing of the past and a laundress was appointed in the mid-century to relieve the sisters from doing the washing, and special night watchers were introduced. London was growing fast, racked with infectious diseases, and the Governors put on record their appreciation of the devoted work of the nursing staff during epidemics of cholera and typhoid.

As Winifred Hector commented at the conclusion of her article, when the nineteenth century opened, the conditions for patients and staff in hospitals like 'Barts' could have given no hint of the revolutionary changes which were to come. It was a long time before the Hospital took on its modern role, and at the beginning of the twentieth century the Hospital still had the distinct social role that looked back to medieval times. At Christmas, even until the mid-twentieth century, ward sisters usually had a list of old patients who looked forward to admission not because they were ill, but because they were lonely and poor. Demand for medical and nursing care in hospital can never be fully satisfied, and the number of beds and the number of nursing staff progressively increased.

Winifred Hector quotes the description from a surgeon who recalled an instance of plastic surgery in pre-anaesthetic days:

> It was on a girl who had been desperately burned on the neck and shoulders by falling into a fire ... She was a repulsive spectacle, and had gladly consented to Mr. Skey's suggestion of an operation, which by transplanting a piece of skin from her arm and dissecting up the cicatrix, appeared to afford some chance of mitigating her unfortunate appearance. The patient was tied to the operating table, as was customary in those days, but before many minutes of the operating had elapsed, her cries and entreaties to be untied, and allowed to remain as she was, were the most frightful that can be imagined. As the operation, which was necessarily a long and slow one, proceeded, her cries became more terrible; first one and then another student fainted, and ultimately all but a determined few had left the theatre, unable to stand the distressing scene.

Another quote is from an elderly nurse recalling, in 1891, one operating theatre which had been used in those earlier times: It still contained the table on which formerly the patients were strapped for operation, before the use of anaesthetic. The cupboards were antiquated; there was one containing sand and when the surgeon felt the floor getting sticky, he called for this and the nurse took a shovelful from the cupboard and spread it on the floor. Another cupboard contained hooks, above which were painted the revered names of well-known surgeons and, on those hooks, they used to hang their discarded society frock-coats – only now fit for operating in. I remember Sir Thomas Smith going to the cupboard to look at the names on the hooks ... and saying how proud Mr. Paget was of his when it became a mahogany colour.

One of the great doctors of the time was James Paget. Surgeon and physiologist, he is considered to be one of the founders of pathology. He worked at St Bartholomew's Hospital between 1834 and 1871 where, as professor of anatomy and surgery, he made many important medical discoveries. In 1875, he became president of the Royal College of Surgeons. As a doctor of international repute, he served as surgeon to Queen Victoria and worked with Ethel Manson and her predecessor Maria Machin, taking a great interest in the development of nursing. He also achieved the impressive feat of managing to be a friend to the great opposing forces of Florence Nightingale and to Ethel Manson.

James Paget was far from satisfied with conditions he found in hospital medicine, as excerpts from letters to his brother record:

> 1836. a case of rheumatic pericarditis ... the man was heavily bled – to 50oz – and died, I should say, of exhaustion ... I wanted to examine [post mortem] ... with a microscope ... and there was none in the hospital.

As was usual practice at the time, Paget and his wife lived within St Bartholomew's Hospital premises. Later, his wife could never forget the cries coming from the operating theatre, a few yards from her home. She firmly maintained that, after the discovery of anaesthesia, in the middle of the century, a day should have been set aside for national thanksgiving.

The science of refrigeration was perfected and in 1880 Australia was able to send a cargo of refrigerated meat to the English markets transported on the SS *Strathleven*. Two years later, SS *Dunedin* brought the first shipment of frozen meat from New Zealand. Refrigeration was to play an important role in commerce, in community health and within hospitals and laboratories as well as eventually within the home.

Ethel Manson achieved the prestigious post of Matron at St Bartholomew's Hospital at a time of development and change and she began to play her part in ensuring it would be change for the better.

# Chapter 4

# The Matron 1881–1887

Nursing was now being perceived as a noble calling. Admiration for Florence Nightingale's well publicised work in the Crimea had resulted in the raising of a testimonial fund, which she had used to start a nurses' training school. This first nurses' school had been started in 1860 at St Thomas's Hospital London and Florence Nightingale, constantly stressing her belief in the vocational aspect of nursing, wrote revealingly in 1889: 'When very many years ago I planned a future, my one idea was not organising a hospital but organising a religion.'

Probationers in her Nightingale school were expected to be punctual at all times when attending lectures, meals, going on duty, attending prayers, and going to bed. They were not to visit each other's rooms after evening prayers. Lights had to be out by 10.30 pm and no baths were permitted after that time. They were expected to be neat and orderly, their rooms always had to have the window open at the top and beds well aired. They were to dress quietly when out of doors, with no flowers, coloured feathers, or hats. Boots, high heeled shoes, fringes, and dress-improvers were not considered appropriate. The probationers were permitted to go out on alternate Sundays to church, but not to visit friends and certainly were not expected to go out alone in the evening. The probationers were expected to keep a diary of their work and their thoughts, which Miss Nightingale would read and comment on in the hopes of checking on and improving their moral characters.

All these strict convent-style rules conformed to the conventions of the age and the vocational perception of nursing. Despite some of the distressing work they undertook, these rules were considered necessary to protect the vulnerable young females. Women were not responsible enough to vote so could not possibly be responsible enough to organise their own lives in the dangerous world outside the hospital. They were, however, expected to be responsible for the conditions and the lives of the patients in their care. Total and absolute dedication was required, with no allowances made for any other distracting interests or private life.

St Bartholomew's School of Nursing was founded in 1877. In 1881, the young Ethel Gordon Manson left her post as Sister in the London Hospital, Whitechapel, and was appointed to the post of Matron of the prestigious St Bartholomew's hospital. A job description of a Matron's duties of the time – much abbreviated – includes the following:

> You shall have the charge, governance, and order of the Sisters, Night Superintendents, Nurses and all other females employed in the Departments under your control. You shall have the direct supervision of the Trained Nurse's Institution. You shall visit every ward in the hospital at least four times a week for the purpose of seeing that the several persons employed therein are strictly performing their respective duties, and that the comfort of the patients is duly cared for, that the Wards and everything appertaining thereto are clean and wholesome, that the regulations for the well governing of the Wards are obeyed and that sobriety, good order, and decorum do prevail therein. You shall take care that every Ward is supplied with a proper staff of efficient Nurses … in cases of emergency, such extra nurses as may be necessary are also provided without delay … in order that the directions of the Physicians and Surgeons with reference to the treatment of their patients may be duly obeyed … you shall be at all times accessible to the Medical and Surgical Officers; and whilst seeing, as far as possible, that their instructions are carried into effect by the Sisters and Nurses, you shall be careful not to interfere with any directions they may have given as regards individual patients, or the management of the Ward so far as it affects the treatment of the patients. You shall exercise a

special oversight of the Probationary Nurses during their period of training, seeing that their work in the Wards is duly supervised by the Sisters …You shall be in frequent communication with the Night Superintendents … you shall require them to make to you every morning a report in writing of any irregularities or other special circumstances which may have some under their notice during the preceding night. You shall see that the Sisters and Nurses and others under your control, to whom leave of absence from their duties may have been granted, do not remain out after the time appointed for their return …You shall exercise a general supervision of the Nurses' home …You shall prepare and certify the Sisters', Nurses' and Female Servants' Wages lists and deliver them to the Clerk's Office on the Monday preceding the day of meeting of the Committee for passing such lists. You shall, every Thursday, make a report in writing to the Treasurer and Almoners of the general condition of your department …With the help of Assistant Matron you shall have charge of all blankets, sheets, materials or liveries for the Female Staff, and all other linen, cotton and stuff goods provided for use in the Hospital; and you shall issue the same from time to time to the several Wards or persons entitled thereto in accordance with the orders of the Governors. But, before the issue of any worn stock, you shall take care that all old or worn-out articles, for which a new issue is to be made, are returned to you. And you shall not issue any new articles to replace articles missing until a statement of the latter has been laid before the Treasurer and Almoners and the proposed issue has been sanctioned by them. You shall keep accounts in books provided for the purpose, of all articles received from the several tradesmen, and of the distribution thereof. You shall occupy such residence or apartments as shall, from time to time, be allotted to you, and not harbour nor receive therein any inmate or lodger. You shall do all such other business respecting this Hospital as the Governors shall assign or appoint; and devote the whole of your time, with diligence and fidelity, to the service of the Hospital, considering yourself as placed in a situation of very great responsibility. You shall on no account sleep away from the Hospital or absent yourself from your duties, without the consent of the Treasurer, or of two almoners in case of his absence, nor shall you, under ordinary circumstances be absent on leave from the Hospital at the same time as the Clerk.

Ethel Manson's predecessor as Matron of St Bartholomew's was Maria Machin, a protégé of Florence Nightingale, who had previously endured a rather unsuccessful time as Matron of the Montreal General Hospital, after which she had then been 'now inclined to seek some work less responsible for a while'. She certainly had selected the wrong post when she went to St Bartholomew's, and she was soon bemoaning to her friend Miss Nightingale that, whenever she wanted to make a change, the Sisters 'signified that they have been accustomed to doing so-and-so' – a not unusual reply from such a tradition-orientated group and still frequently heard today throughout the hospital wards!

Miss Machin had hoped to instil the principles of the Nightingale School into St Bartholomew's and to this end brought some of the Nightingale-trained nurses who had worked with her in Canada to fill vacant Sisters' posts. She succeeded in raising the minimum age for probationers from 20 to 23 and increased the length of training from one year to two.

In 1880, William Savory, one of the surgeons, informed Florence Nightingale that Miss Machin had improved the character of the probationary nurses and that their work had become more satisfactory. James Paget, his senior colleague, said that she was well esteemed by all the medical staff and told Florence Nightingale that 'the changes already made for the better are far more than could have been expected ten or fifteen years ago'.

However, Paget, wisely counselled caution, foreseeing the problems and opposition that could occur if she tried to act too quickly. As he feared, Miss Machin became impatient because of her inability to make change as rapidly as she wished. The influence of her Nightingale training meant that, although she had a strong sense of vocation, she lacked managerial skills. She complained how little she had been able to achieve after almost a year in office and wrote with frustration, 'The Hospital authorities prefer gradual improvement to radical reforms.'

Understandably, the untrained Sisters were obstructive towards sudden new ideas and she could not persuade them to change their traditional ways. Compounding her problems, the hospital Treasurer was often too busy to see her. Exasperated, Miss Machin sent her letter of resignation in January 1881 after little more than two frustrating years as Matron.

The hospital records show that in 1880 a total of 6,314 patients were treated in St Bartholomew's – 586 of them died. Just over 600 patients were schoolchildren and there were three cases of malaria, 109 cases of typhoid – of which nineteen died, and nine out of the fourteen diphtheria patients died. Tuberculosis accounted for eighty-seven patients of whom thirty-six died and six out of seven women with puerperal fever died. One note in the records is somewhat alarming: 'In one case symptoms resembling those of enteric fever were accounted for in the discovery of more than one dead cat in the cistern which supplied the drinking water.'

By its charter the hospital was only permitted to nurse the sick poor. Patients came from an area of London where there were many labourers, carmen, butchers, porters, and printers. As well as the twenty-one gardeners, the twelve grooms nursed there are a reminder that this was the age of the horse-drawn vehicle. The occupations of the female patients reflect the range of work available for women and include laundresses, housewives, charwomen, machinists, needlewomen, cooks, shop-women, hawkers, ironers, and 137 harlots. Unsurprisingly, the recorded twelve female lead-carriers all had lead poisoning.

Ethel Gordon Manson started as Matron of 'Barts' in the spring of 1881 and set out to make immediate improvements. Her appointment may perhaps be seen as a conscious decision by St Bartholomew's to break with the Nightingale tradition. Twenty-four-year-old Ethel Manson was almost certainly the youngest Matron the Hospital has ever had and some of the senior medical staff objected to her appointment on the grounds that she was too young and too attractive. However, having already received good reports of her, Sir Sydney Waterlow had paid discreet visits to her ward at the London Hospital to inspect her methods of working. He was impressed by her character that was undaunted by difficulties, by her determination, and her abilities. At her interview, she convinced the Treasurer that she was not afraid of anyone and would be quite capable of managing the old Sisters.

Ethel Manson was initially appointed for a trial period of six months, but in December 1881 Sir Sidney Waterlow reported to the Governors that she had been found highly suitable. The new Matron was consequently confirmed in her post with an initial salary of £250 per annum. Ethel was determined to succeed, and in later years she was remembered as someone who had swept through the Hospital like a whirlwind.

The needs of the patients were paramount, but Ethel understood that unfit and overtired nurses cannot fulfil those needs adequately – she understood that nurses themselves need care. There was much to be done and, as the new Matron, Ethel adjusted some of the worst features of the nurses' working hours, improved the food by raising the protein level, and constantly asked the Governors for salary increases for old servants and those with special responsibilities. She visited each ward in turn every day, devoting three hours every morning and two hours every evening to ensuring that cleanliness and efficiency were maintained.

Things had improved greatly since Florence Nightingale had reported, after visiting overcrowded hospital wards, in the 1840s, 'It was common practice to put a patient into the same sheets used by the last occupants of the bed, and mattresses were of flock, seldom, if ever, cleaned.' Where she found old and unnecessary practices, such as getting patients out of bed before 6.00 am, or making them help with bedmaking, Ethel Manson insisted that these be discontinued. As she recorded in the *British Journal of Nursing* on 4 July 1903, 'I owe that where duty was concerned, I was a somewhat exacting taskmistress. I was young and an enthusiast ... sixteen hours work made up a normal day. Ease, unpunctuality, omissions, short measure of work – these were unpardonable crimes.'

In contrast to the common belief that 'good nurses are born not made', Ethel understood that it was not enough for a nurse to be a gentle and empathetic 'ministering angel'. A good nurse must have self-discipline and a wealth of knowledge gained from education. She also believed that, in order to understand the needs of patients who came from all walks of life, a nurse must be aware of events outside medicine and appreciate that the world was bigger than the narrow confines of the ward.

Ethel demanded the highest standards from her nurses, but was also an indefatigable campaigner for improvements in their training and working conditions, achieving improvements in their food and obtaining increased off-duty hours and holidays for them. That she was no administration handmaiden or lackey is evident from her emphatic instruction – 'always support nurses against Doctors and administrators'.

After her arrival at 'Barts', she endorsed and improved the probationer trial system, whereby candidates were accepted for training only after working for at least one month as 'extra nurses'. During her first month in post, a structured teaching plan was introduced and detailed reports on the progress of all probationers were started. In their first year, probationers worked in different wards in rotation, spending three months in each of four wards to gain experience.

St Bartholomew's had begun to train nurses in 1877 and originally nurse training had been for a year. By 1879, this had been extended to two years, but Ethel Manson increased the training further. In 1882, examinations were held at the end of the first year and the course was then extended to three years. Practical work was interspersed with theoretical instruction. As well as enlarging the sphere of work and improving the probationers' knowledge, this was also an ideal way in which to increase the number of nurses on the wards as the workload became more complex and demanding.

When they became newly qualified, the probationers were encouraged to become staff nurses and, as the majority of the older nursing staff had been given no formal training, this new input gradually built up the contingent of trained nurses. With the major expansion of medical and surgical knowledge, it was eventually possible for nurses to lay claim to a specific or specialised body of work and responsibility for their patients.

As a disciplinarian and a reformer, Ethel Manson was determined that her high standards should be reflected in the uniforms worn by her staff. Very aware of the importance of appearance, she understood that outward neatness projected professional efficiency. In the 1870s, uniform was haphazard, caps and aprons worn – or not – according to individual fancy. Miss Manson wanted every Sister to be dressed with military precision, with not a button out of place. She is reputed to have personally measured every yard of cap frilling to ensure that it was exactly correct.

Previously the Sisters had worn blue merino wool dresses without caps or aprons, but the pattern was left to the Sisters' discretion. Miss Manson persuaded all the Sisters to wear an identical uniform and asked the Hospital to supply frilly caps and strapless aprons – 'for such of the Sisters as were willing to wear them'. Another change was the uniform of the staff nurses; the old brown dresses were phased out because the trained nurses objected to wearing them. In 1881, she introduced caps of a standard design to be worn by all nurses. The certified nurses and the second and third-year probationers were given a uniform of blue and white striped material instead of the plain grey of the first-year probationers. Staff nurses wore a blue belt, the second-year and third-year probationers a white one. Like the Sisters, nurses had caps with strings tied under the chin, but their aprons were of different design with straps at the shoulders.

Miss Manson began to recruit a new type of nurse. Twenty-six probationers from widely varied backgrounds started their training in her first year in office. Twelve gave London addresses, ten came from the English provinces, one from Wales, two from Scotland, and one from the Netherlands. Six had some kind of previous nursing experience, seven had been in domestic service, and one was formerly a teacher in a Board School. Others were evidently from middle-class families and two candidates had been employed as governesses. There were also several young ladies in their twenties who had no previous work experience. The Hospital was willing to train girls from any background, humble or otherwise, as long as they could meet the right standards.

Three years after arriving at St Bartholomew's, Ethel Manson introduced a scheme for a different type of nurse. Paying Probationers, in groups of twelve to fifteen, were educated young women who wished to gain some practical knowledge of nursing. They could become 'special probationers' for a period of three months and were known as 'ladies' in order to distinguish them from the other candidates. Similar schemes already existed in other London hospitals, but Barts was unique in calling them 'special probationers'. The scheme was very popular and many of the 'ladies' asked for an extension of another three months. Their presence was perceived as a good influence and also allowed the regular staff to have more time off-duty. The scheme attracted many applicants, women of the educated class who, it was presumed, did not need the meagre salaries of the ordinary probationer and did not want to commit themselves to three whole years of hard work on the wards. Sir James Paget found the scheme successful and remarked that in his youth the admission of young ladies to be nurses in this or any other similar hospital would have been thought scandalous, yet in the event proved wholly acceptable.

The special probationers did not live with the other nurses, but had separate accommodation in King Square, Finsbury. They were excused night duty, and came on duty at 8.00 am or 8.30 am instead of 7.00 am. In spite of these privileges, every special probationer was left in no doubt that strict punctuality and obedience were required of them. They had to adhere to the strict set of rules which included no writing letters, receiving friends, reading novels or doing fancy work while they were on duty. The wearing of jewellery or high heels and curled or fringed hairstyles were forbidden. In spite of these strictures and the hard work, many of the special probationers were determined to carry on nursing and after three months they chose to stay on as ordinary probationers. Eventually St Bartholomew's was recognised as the most socially acceptable hospital for young ladies to train, and girls with fathers ranging from merchants to dukes were eager to join its ranks of nurses.

Each week, Miss Manson wrote a catalogue of illness and infections amongst her staff in a report to the Treasurer and the Almoners. These records show the wastage rate from each nurses' school, and the reasons for withdrawal. The probationers suffered complaints including bad backs, delicate health, and feet too swollen to stand upon. Amongst the illnesses are sore throats, erysipelas, rheumatic fever, nephritis, diphtheria, and typhoid. A Sister Radcliffe died of typhus in 1882 and a Nurse Godolphin-Osborne had one joint after another amputated from a septic finger, until she lost the whole finger. In the days before antibiotics, this was not an uncommon occurrence for nurses who changed septic dressings regularly. Bearing in mind the many incurable diseases of the time, it is remarkable that so many young girls did survive working such long and arduous hours in such a dangerous environment.

The experience she gained as Matron soon convinced Ethel Manson of the need for professional independence in nursing. The public had no protection against women who called themselves nurses but who had no training, and there was also a lack of protection and support for trained nurses. She persuaded the hospital authorities that the ward assistants should be given a three-year contract. This would prevent them leaving after one year, pronouncing themselves nurses, and taking nursing posts in other hospitals.

Hospitals frequently supplied trained nurses for private cases, some such as the London Hospital sending out probationers as 'trained' nurses. This was a time when surgical operations were often performed in the home, with nurses instructed how to prepare a room for these operations, and the practice continued for many years. Ethel Manson deplored this use of probationers as being deceptive and in 1886 she started a Trained Nurses Institute at St Bartholomew's. Private nurses were often exploited by employers, their fee being paid to the hospital's private institution, and to counteract this Ethel Manson ensured that these nurses – usually employed for maternity or for massage cases – received their fee directly.

Broadening of knowledge and increased availability of treatment gave a nurse the opportunity to take over more control of patient care. A great development was in 1887 when ready-made sterile wrapped and sealed surgical dressings were manufactured. Nurses were now responsible for the patients' environment, provision of comfort, care before, during and after operation, observation of signs and symptoms, sterilisation of equipment, and prevention of spread of infection. No longer just a handmaiden, the nurse had developed into a skilled colleague with her own specialties to offer the medical team.

The suggestion that nurses should be registered had been made by Dr Henry Ackland in 1874 in a preface to *A Handbook for Hospital Sisters* by Miss Florence Lees. However, the proposed register (to indicate a nurse had received a prescribed training before reaching a specified level of competence) was not a popular suggestion. It was generally believed that moral character rather than technical ability was more important and that a national standard was irrelevant.

Following their own struggles for professional registration, the British Medical Association always supported the nurses' registration scheme. Sadly, the main objectors were within the ranks of nurses themselves. Although admitting that in fifty years' time the idea might just be feasible, Florence Nightingale was the most formidable opponent of registration and she found the increasing activism divisive and disturbing.

Ethel had acquired an impressive reputation, as is evident from a newspaper article of the time:

> Miss Manson, whose charming manner and appearance will still be remembered in Nottingham, is earning for herself a marvelous reputation in the profession of nursing. Miss Manson began her

training as a probationer in the Children's Hospital in Nottingham some eight years ago. She is now lady superintendent of nursing at St. Bartholomew's Hospital, London, has charge of 670 beds, and has lately been presented with a beautifully engraved testimonial for services rendered, signed by H.R.H. Princess of Wales, as President of the National Health Exhibition. She has also been honoured by being unanimously elected as a representative of nursing and domestic arrangement by the Council of the Hospital Association, and by having been requested to deliver a course of lectures on the 'Art of Nursing' by H.R.H. Princess Christian. We feel sure that she will benefit and delight her audience, as she speaks with charming distinctness and fluency, and has been heard to recite with rare power and pathos.

A few days later, a report of the first lecture appeared in the paper.

A crowded audience assembled at the residence of the Hon. Mrs. Jenne, Wimpole Street, W. on the 30th ult., to listen to the first of a series of three lectures on 'Nursing' given under the auspices of the National Health Society by Miss Manson, Matron of St. Bartholomew's Hospital. The lecturer, whose youth aroused some surprise among her audience, who remembered the importance of her post at the head of the nursing staff at one of the largest of London hospitals, wore her professional costume, consisting of a plain black robe, with white headdress, collar, and cuffs. She took for her subject 'The Development of the Art of Nursing', and in recommending her lecture asked the indulgence of her hearers, on the grounds that it was her first appearance in public. Indulgence, however, was by no means needed, the lecturer's voice being musical, her utterance clear, and the literary style of her composition excellent. Miss Manson referred to the earliest hospitals in pre-Christian times, pointing out how hospitals for animals as well as men formerly existed in India, how in Greece rooms were set aside in the Temple of Aesculapius for the sick, who came to worship at his shrine. No hospitals, which could be properly so called, existed in Europe, however, until Christianity became the religion of the Latin state; the great hospital of Basil was endowed by the Emperor Valentian. In 850 the Council of Padua relegated the care of the sick to the Church, in whose hands it remained for many centuries. From the earliest times among the German races medicine and surgery were entirely in the hands of women, and it was not until monasteries became general that men took their part in the art of healing. The Hospital of St Bernard, still justly famous, was founded in 980, but most of the many hospitals nursed by knightly and religious orders in the Middle Ages were devoted to the care of lepers. When in the fourteenth and fifteenth centuries leprosy gradually died out, these leper houses became general hospitals. A Mussulman hospital was established on a grand scale at Cairo in 1283, the patients being well cared for. In after years however, hospitals became mere pest houses, the patients being neglected and starved, so that the officials might make larger incomes. In 1784, at the Hotel Dieu in Paris, there was only one bed for every twelve patients, six lying on the floor whilst the others were in bed, and afterwards changing with them. Going onto the history of her own hospital, Miss Manson stated that St. Bartholomew's Hospital was founded in 1123 by Rayher, the minstrel of Henry II who was visited by a vision of the saint, who demanded that the hospital should be named after him. Rayher worked with a staff consisting of a master, eight brothers, and three sisters. The hospital was nursed by the Augustinian Order until the Reformation, when its care, with that of similar institutions, passed from the Church to civic authorities, and St. Bartholomew's then has a staff of matron and twelve nurses for one hundred patients. In 1557 a code of comprehensive rules was drawn up, many of which rules are still in force. In later times the name of hospital and nurse became blotted, and Sarah Gamp and her congeners ruled the day.

From that degradation of the art nursing was rescued by Florence Nightingale, and women of talent and refinement now find their vocation as nurses. Miss Manson concluded with a touching and poetical picture of the sort of woman an ideal nurse should be, and strongly censured those who enter the profession from sordid motives, or because they are unsuited for social life. At the end of this interesting and eloquent lecture Mr. Cripps, a member of the medical staff of St. Bartholomew's Hospital, proposed a vote of thanks to Miss Manson.

Ethel was part of a new wave of nursing, determined that the nurse could no longer be perceived as being like the drunken Sairey Gamp, caricatured by Charles Dickens, and bribeable with offerings of gin. Most occupations for women were oversubscribed and nursing was no exception. It was now seen as a respectable occupation and in spite of the long hours, poor conditions, and dangers, it began to attract more educated women than could be trained. Some years later, when giving evidence to a Select Committee of the House of Lords, Ethel Manson stated: 'The last year I was at St. Bartholomew's I had one thousand five hundred letters of inquiry. I do not call them applications ... but letters of inquiry for, say, fifty vacancies.'

Ethel Manson instigated many reforms and improvements for the benefit of both patients and of nurses. She was determined to see St Bartholomew's staffed entirely with trained nurses. By the time she left the Hospital, most of the untrained Sisters and nurses had been weeded out, although a few of the better ones remained in office – the last untrained Sister not retiring until 1907. This new policy meant that there were many promotion opportunities for the best of the qualified nurses. A good example is that of the first gold medallist, Hannah Turner, who was made a Ward Sister within two months of completing her training. By the time Ethel Manson left St Bartholomew's, the excellent reputation of the training course was well known and there was no shortage of applicants

In 1881, Louis Pasteur demonstrated a means of immunisation against anthrax, by injection of a comparatively harmless culture of the bacillus causing that disease. From then on, widespread and intensive searches for new vaccines began.

Research into disease-causing micro-organisms had proved challenging until Angelina Hesse provided the answer. Angelina's husband Walther was a laboratory assistant for Robert Koch, one of the founders of microbiology and, as well as illustrating his publications, Angelina helped her husband prepare growth mediums. Researchers had struggled to isolate and grow bacteria on a variety of mediums, including potatoes, wheat, egg whites, and eventually gelatine but, unfortunately, gelatine liquified at the temperature most suitable for the growth of bacteria. Amongst her many other accomplishments, Angelina was also a cook, and had learnt about the properties of an ingredient used to set jellies in hot climates – agar-agar. She suggested this would be suitable for their research and it proved to be the ideal medium for cultivating cultures of bacteria. Consequently, in 1882, Dr Robert Koch was able to announce to the world that he had isolated the organism responsible for tuberculosis. The contribution made by Angelina Hesse was not acknowledged and she received no reward for a discovery which is still of benefit in medicinal research today.

Irish protesters began a terror campaign while, in 1883, Britain occupied Egypt. Massive dust clouds from the eruption of the volcano of Krakatoa resulted in spectacular red sunsets for weeks in Britain during the late summer of 1883.

A revolt against British rule in the Sudan resulted in the siege of Khartoum. In Britain, in December 1884, a Parliamentary Reform Act opened the franchise to all adult males, with the exception of domestic servants, bachelors living with their parents, and those of no fixed address. Following a third Anglo-Burmese war, Britain finally annexed Burma. The first British labour exchanges were established in 1885 and the first cremation of modern times took place in Woking crematorium in March that year.

Ethel's stepfather, George Storer, had been re-elected as Member of Parliament in 1880 but his tenure as a Conservative MP ended in 1885, when his constituency was abolished by the Redistribution of Seats Act in 1885. Local newspapers recorded that he had been an indefatigable MP. His staunch protection of the rural economy in his support of the taxation of imports is recorded in Hansard. One of his early speeches had been concerning the repeal of the malt tax, during which he revealed that his wife was one of the best brewers in the county.

Parliamentary upheavals continued; following a hostile reception to his budget, William Gladstone resigned and Conservative Lord Salisbury became Prime Minister once again.

Four years after demonstrating a means of immunisation against anthrax, Louis Pasteur developed a vaccine for rabies. Wilhelm Rontgen, a German physicist, had seen the powers of X-rays in 1885 when he was able to reveal an image of the bones in his wife's hand on a photographic plate. Seeds of further changes were being sown when, in 1886, Elsie Inglis entered the newly opened Edinburgh School of medicine, which was run by another medical pioneer, Sophia Jex-Blake. The name of Elsie Inglis was to be well known in the years ahead.

Psychiatry was unheard of at this time, and patients with mental illness were often hidden and abandoned in institutions. In America, Nellie Bly, a newspaper reporter, feigned insanity in order to investigate conditions in a mental asylum. Her writings about the patients who were being subjected to neglect and violence eventually resulted in nationwide reform.

By 1886, gold was discovered in the Transvaal and with the increasing exploitation of diamonds, South Africa became the main jewel in the Imperial crown, encouraging waves of entrepreneurs to seek their fortunes in that new continent. The Dutch Voortreckers had already penetrated much of the country and in their wanderings had been forced to become medically self-sufficient. They had discovered and used more than 100 different types of new plants from the veldt, including the now popular aloe. Some of their medical practices appeared bizarre, although nowadays it is possible to understand why an application of cobwebs and sugar to an open wound could well be effective. The Boers were very aware of the importance of not polluting their water source and, due to a combination of hardiness, common-sense and adaptability, managed to survive well in their hostile environment.

Time was becoming more important in a busy developing world and in 1885 GMT was adopted as the meridian of a system for international standard time. A Canadian, Sandford Fleming, had conceived and developed the system, which divided the world into twenty-four time zones, with standard time in each zone.

In 1883, British troops had been used to suppress crofter demonstrations on the Isle of Skye. A law passed in 1886 finally gave security of tenure to crofters and an end to the iniquitous Highland Clearances. This law resulted in the resignation from the Cabinet of the Duke of Argyll in protest at such infringement of what he considered to be his rights as a landowner.

In 1886, a German, von Bergmann, introduced steam sterilisation, which would change and improve hospital practices immeasurably. The development of steam sterilisation of dressings and equipment was a major advancement in patient care. Once those techniques had been introduced, generations of night nurses, listening to the snores and groans of dozing patients, would huddle around the ward table under the desk-light, trying not to sneeze as they carefully filled the sterilising drums with individually rolled cotton wool balls and gauze swabs for the next day's dressing round. The instrument drum would be packed with metal and glass syringes, ancient scissors and forceps. Each individual injection needle would be carefully inspected to ensure the point was not bent or hooked before sealing it into the drum for sterilisation and re-use. The filled drums would be collected and taken to the great steam sterilising machines before being sealed and returned to the wards. Metal instruments and bowls would be boiled during the night in the ward sterilisers and laid out carefully for the morning dressing round. These techniques were at the forefront of infection control up until the

1960s. Thanks to her contacts throughout the medical and nursing world, Ethel played a role in helping to introduce them to British hospital wards, thereby reducing infection rates in the era before antibiotics.

Although many things were beginning to change, there remained massive social divisions in Britain. Society life consisted of endless rounds of dinner parties and formal engagements – functions far removed from the harsh realities of the rest of the world. It was the age of the chaperone and the social round, with strict etiquette being of vital importance. Scandal was avoided at all costs, not simply by good behaviour, but often by the expedient of turning a blind eye and hushing things up. Most young society gentlemen had mistresses so that, when they married, they had a second establishment to pension off or to maintain.

In London, in the late afternoons, the riding track along the south side of Hyde Park, known as Rotten Row, was the place to see and be seen. State carriages and barouches were pulled up under the trees with the beautifully dressed occupants gracefully acknowledging the salutations of gentlemen who raised their hats in passing. High-stepping horses drew phaetons while their passengers indulged in gossip, met friends, and made appointments and assignations.

The other side of Victorian society was dark and dismal; poverty, starvation, and disease ran rampant. Typical were London match girls, born in slums, who were driven to work while still children. Undersized because they were underfed, they worked a twelve-hour day in appalling and dangerous conditions and under harsh discipline. If they became sick or ill, they received no wages and they were discarded when they were worked out. The ageing Poet Laureate, Lord Tennyson, highlighted the problems:

> Is it well that while we range with Science, glorying in the Time
> City children soak and blacken soul and sense in city slime?
> There among the glooming alleys Progress halts on palsied feet
> Crime and hunger cast out maidens by the thousand on the street,
> There the Master scrimps his haggard seamstress of her daily bread,

There a single sordid attic holds the living and the dead.
There the smoldering fire of fever creeps across the rotted floor,
And the crowded couch of incest in the warrens of the poor.

The squalor of places such as Whitechapel provided ideal conditions for disease and crime, allowing psychopaths such as Jack the Ripper to flourish. However, social awareness and a sense of social responsibility were developing and began to take a political form. The Fabian Society became more prominent as the realisation grew that, in spite of great industrial advances, many people had been left behind in workless squalor.

The 'Bloody Sunday' riot in Trafalgar Square in November 1887 proved that all was not well. Public figures such Bernard Shaw, H. G. Wells, and Sydney and Beatrice Webb became recognised as social evolutionists. Another visionary was the young Ramsay MacDonald, future Labour Prime Minister, who had been born in Moray, just a few short miles away from Ethel Manson's birthplace.

Ahead of its time, a pneumatic wheel had been patented as early as 1845 but it was left to John B. Dunlop, a British veterinary surgeon, to found the tyre industry by patenting and developing pneumatic tyres for bicycles and tricycles in 1888. His work had a great influence on popularising cycling, both as a hobby and as a means of transport, and by the end of the century solid rubber tyres were being manufactured for horse-drawn carriages.

The bicycle was becoming popular and the new 'safety' bicycle was offering unimagined freedom to adventurous women. There had been a lot of enraged controversy about the propriety of a 'lady' riding a bicycle. Revealing any amount of leg was a frightful disgrace – a woman's leg supposedly a thing known only to herself and God. Women were liberating themselves from the tyranny of the corset and voluminous skirts and, once the cross bar was dropped, more women took up cycling. A young lady recalled how her long skirt was a danger and she found herself constantly tumbling onto the cobbles with her skirt wrapped so tightly around the pedal that she could hardly get up to unwrap it. In spite of this problem, she lacked the courage to ride in breeches, except at night – although knickerbockers were being worn with aplomb by daring Frenchwomen. In America, by the 1890s, the women's reformer Amelia Jenks Bloomer advocated more rational dress for women. She gave her name to a highly contentious garment which was enthusiastically embraced by pioneering women cyclists.

In Battersea Park, London, people could be seen exhibiting their bicycling prowess by solemnly peddling up and down. In the shady pathways, the less experienced wobbled and battled persistently with gravity and cycling instructors guaranteed proficiency in twelve lessons. One society lady employed two footmen to walk alongside to prop her up while she tried to master her machine. Women cyclists were subjected to much harassment and criticism from men who did not approve of such displays of independence. Cabmen would converge from behind on a female cyclist, omnibus drivers would flick them with their whip and boisterous lads would link hands across the road in front of them, presenting a daunting obstruction to the intrepid pedaller. Despite these challenges, on experiencing a hitherto unknown freedom to travel independently, women delighted in this new form of transport and the bicycle was soon to prove a vital means of transport for many district nurses and midwives.

At that time, it was not considered possible for a woman to carry on with her nursing career once she married. Ethel Manson was dedicated to her career, but eventually succumbed to the charms of tall and handsome Dr Bedford Fenwick, who she had worked with at the London Hospital.

Dr Bedford Fenwick held several appointments at the London Hospital and, amongst his other duties at the London Hospital, had also achieved the distinction of becoming the royal gynaecologist. Eldest son of Sam Fenwick, a doctor from North Shields, he was one of two sisters and five brothers. All of his brothers had medical careers, were all professionally excellent and, as specialists, they passed patients on to one another. However, years later Ethel's grandson recalled that frequent quarrels and intrigues meant that the brothers were never socially all on speaking terms at the same time.

Despite her strong admiration for the dashing Dr Bedford Fenwick, the Matron of the London, Eva Luckes, had not succeeded in winning his deeper affection. Later, within the family, the story was told that Ethel only agreed to marry the persistent doctor if he could cure a particular seriously ill patient. Dr Bedford Fenwick successfully took up her challenge, the patient recovered and, in 1887 at the age of 30, Ethel resigned her post in order to marry.

From Matron Ethel Manson, St Bartholomew's inherited a commitment to a three-year professional training and a belief that nursing was a career for intelligent women of any social class. Her friend and successor, Isla Stewart, also took up this cause, and the Hospital became a bastion in the struggle for registration.

In 1887, the *Morning Post* carried the announcement: 'The marriage arranged between Dr. Bedford Fenwick and Miss Ethel Gordon Manson will take place at the Church of St. Bartholomew-the-Less, West Smithfield on Wednesday, the 6th July at two o'clock.'

Despite the conventions of the time, marriage was not to be the end of Ethel's nursing career.

## Chapter 5

# Celebrations, Marriage, and New Challenges 1887–1899

The year Ethel married, 1887, was one of other, very public, celebrations. It was Queen Victoria's Golden Jubilee, marking the fiftieth year of her reign. In Calcutta, all the ladies ordered 'Jubilee bustles' and in London streets and houses were decorated with flags, banners, fairy lights, and paper lanterns to celebrate the great event.

On Jubilee Day, 21 June 1887, over 600 peers and peeresses, seated uncomfortably on narrow benches, attended a celebratory ceremony in Westminster Abbey. The following day, over 30,000 children enjoyed a school treat in Hyde Park and were provided with a bag containing a meat-pie, a bun, and an orange as well as a Jubilee mug of Doulton-ware. Later in the afternoon, the Life Guards headed a great procession of royalty and chieftains from all over the world. In the evening, a thousand boys of Eton College put on a torch-light display at Windsor Castle, the smallest boys carrying Chinese lanterns in a winding procession up the hill opposite the Queen's window.

A fund had been established to commemorate the Golden Jubilee and Queen Victoria devoted most of it to the Jubilee Institute for Nurses, founded specifically to nurse the sick poor in their own homes with trained nurses. One of the advisers and trustees of this fund was the ageing Sir James Paget, who met with Florence Nightingale several times in connection with the fund's administration.

The wedding of Ethel Gordon Manson, Matron of St Bartholomew's Hospital, and Dr Bedford Fenwick, eldest son of Dr Fenwick of 29, Harley Street, was well reported in newspapers, including the

# Celebrations, Marriage, and New Challenges 1887–1899

*London Morning Post*. It took place on 6 July 1887 in the Church of St Bartholomew the Less, Smithfield, which had only seen one other such ceremony many years previously. The church had been beautifully decorated with flowers by the nursing staff while, along with her mother and stepfather, Ethel's married sister Clara played a large part in the guest arrangements. The church was filled with hundreds of uniformed nurses and sisters. Family and friends were joined by members of the senior hospital staff and the new Matron, Isla Stewart, was also present.

Noting briefly that the groom wore regulation morning costume with a flower in his buttonhole, the report continued:

> The Church presented a striking show of uniforms and most becoming white caps, while the medical school had to content themselves with places outside the building, where they gave hearty cheers as soon as the bride made her appearance. On each side of the centre aisle rows of nurses, alternate staff, and probationers stood ready with flowers to throw before the bride. Punctually at two o'clock the bride appeared, and Dr. Haberden played the opening bars of a hymn. The choir had been augmented by several members of the medical staff. The bride was given away by her step-father, Mr. Geo. Storer of Thoroton Hall, Notts., and was followed to the altar by her two nieces, Miss Vincent and Miss Aileen Vincent, the daughters of Colonel Arthur Vincent, of Summerhill, county of Limerick, Ireland. They were very prettily dressed in white with straw hats and white feathers. Miss Manson's wedding dress was white striped watered silk, draped with crepe de Chine and a white tulle bonnet was also worn. Her bouquet was magnificent, and much pleasure was felt later on at the sister's dining table when it was found she had paid them the pretty compliment of leaving the bouquet behind for their benefit. When Mr. Swan had duly married the young couple, Mr. Ostle read the Bishop of Bedford's marriage address. As the bride left the altar Wagner's wedding march from 'Lohengrin' was played.

The wedding party then adjourned to a nearby hotel and the report then contained a long list of important wedding guests before continuing: Miss Manson received innumerable presents, and amongst those most valued were four testimonials given to her by her fellow workers at the hospital. Some members of the governing body and medical staff presented a canteen of table silver of the rat-tail pattern. From the sisters and nursing staff came a handsome silver tea and coffee service with kettle, hot water jug, and sugar tongs; From Sister Francis and the Probationers a silver afternoon tea service to match, and a silver inkstand. Fourteen of the late resident medical staff gave four silver candle-sticks, with fittings and lamps complete.

Other gifts included cheques from family members as well as one from the governor of St Bartholomew's. A brief line at the end of the article mentioned that the groom also received 'many handsome and useful wedding presents'!

The newlyweds set up house in 20 Upper Wimpole Street, which was to be Ethel's home until 1924. Once married, Ethel was able to indulge her taste for some luxuries and initially she was unable to resist spending her housekeeping money on antiques and fine porcelain. Her new husband eventually accepted the inevitable, took over the household bills and gave her a personal allowance.

Mrs Bedford Fenwick, as Ethel was now known, went on to begin her thirty-year campaign for state registration of trained nurses. Although, as a married woman, she was not able to remain in her post as Matron, Ethel was now determined to devote her time to the cause of nursing reform. She had already been responsible for helping to improve the standards of nurses and of nursing, but her real work was just beginning. In the fight for recognition of professional standards and registration, Ethel Fenwick could have had no idea how long and how hard a struggle lay ahead.

# Celebrations, Marriage, and New Challenges 1887–1899

In late Victorian England, there were many social divisions. The conventions of society were all-important to the self-preservation of the affluent classes. Their important 'Season' consisted of a set series of events, parties, dinners, balls, and races attended by the select few. At the right age, young girls from upper-class families were presented at court and were said to be 'coming out' into society. They were introduced to the strict rules of etiquette and were displayed at the various social events in an attempt to secure a suitable marriage.

Lady Warwick, a prominent member of Victorian society, reminisced:

> When I came out, social prestige meant something. There was a definite aristocratic Society of the landowning families. These families owned practically the whole of England. It was difficult to enter that Society from the outside, and impossible unless royalty approved. The Prince of Wales was broadish-minded and inclined to welcome some of the professional class. A few artists and doctors were accepted. Sometimes a rich manufacturer might be able to poke his nose in, but he caught it for his temerity no matter how rich he might be. Political people were included, and any outstanding man or woman, say an explorer or a musician, but brains were rarely appreciated and literary people and intellectuals were not welcome. As for newspaper men, their entry was unheard of. Society did not want to be made to think.

These extreme divisions in society were not to last, and the final years of the nineteenth century saw much agitation for change in working conditions throughout the world. People began to demand more reasonable hours and better treatment and, in 1888, Brazil became the last country to officially abolish slavery. An apparently insignificant invention heralded a major change in attitudes to work when Willard L. Bundy invented the time clock, which stamped workers' cards as they reported for work at offices and factories. From then on, time became a resource to be monitored and managed and the race began to do more, to do it ever faster, and for ever greater profits.

America caused worldwide outrage when the death sentence was passed on eight political activists. Fighting for improvements which included an eight-hour day, child protection, and basic safety rights, the American Federation of Labour had organised a peaceful strike in Chicago in 1886. The police reacted fiercely, and the rally culminated in injury and several deaths. Eight protesters, known as the Haymarket Martyrs, were subsequently arrested, tried, and convicted of murder. Four of them were hanged, and public indignation at their sentences resulted in 1 May 1889 being declared a holiday in memory of the dead workers.

Having enjoyed the responsibility and challenges of her work at St Bartholomew's, it was obvious that the new Mrs Fenwick would not sit quietly at home. Shortly after her marriage, and with her husband's support, she opened Gordon House Home Hospital, Holles Street. This eight-bedded private nursing home for surgical patients was newly decorated and comfortably furnished and a qualified cook was employed to ensure suitable, nourishing meals were guaranteed. Ethel employed a few hospital-trained nurses and, giving them further guidance and instructions, trained them up to her superior standards. Here she was able to put into practice her theory that 'sick people could have the scientific nursing of the best hospitals combined with the refinements and luxuries of a well-ordered home.' This new establishment was within easy reach of skilled surgeons and physicians from the West End of London. The charge for a room at this excellent nursing home was between five and eight guineas a week, which included food and nursing. A dedicated individual nurse would cost extra.

Within months of her marriage, Ethel had also started the campaign for registration of trained nurses. She passionately believed in the professionalisation of nursing, understanding the necessity for the regulation of national training followed by examinations to prove competence. A register of these qualified nurses, like the one for doctors, was the only way to attain a professional status and Ethel worked tirelessly to prove her point.

President of the General Medical Council, Dr Henry Acland, had first mentioned registration in 1874, when he emphasised that the medical Act of 1858 allowed women to be registered as medical practitioners but made no provision for the registration of trained nurses. Nursing was a worthwhile career for intelligent, educated, specifically trained individuals and it needed a professional standing which would attract people who were unafraid to be accountable for their professional actions.

Changes within the nursing world progressed slowly. The Hospital Association, founded in 1884 by (later Sir) Henry Burdett, a well-known authority on hospital administration and finance, had discussed registration in 1886, proposing a one-year training scheme. This went totally against the recommendation of the nurse members, who had shown their disapproval by resigning. Ethel Fenwick condemned the scheme as derogatory to nurses and of no value to the public, who would be misled into believing that a nurse with one year of training was competent. The formation of a new group was obviously required.

Isla Stewart, from Moffat, Scotland, was Ethel's close friend, confidant and successor as Matron at St Bartholomew's, and the two women worked together to establish nursing as a properly registered profession. They soon found themselves opposed by the managements of other hospitals, who saw the registration movement as an attack on their powers of control over their nurses. Followers of Florence Nightingale, to whom nursing was a quasi-religious vocation, also disagreed with these new ideas of registration. It was felt that, as long as she was a young lady of good moral character, a nurse only required one or two years of general training.

In November 1887, the new Mrs Fenwick held a meeting in her house at Upper Wimpole Street. A group of hospital matrons, including her friend Isla Stewart, and a number of physicians gathered together to discuss the future organisation of the nursing profession and decided to form an association of nurses.

The newly formed association all agreed that the best protection of trained nurses against untrained women was to establish a register, similar to the doctors' register. The minimum qualification should be three years' training in a hospital. At their second meeting in December, the name 'British Nurses' Association' was adopted. Several matrons who had resigned from the Hospital Association became the founders of the British Nurses' Association. From then on, with this group behind her, Mrs Bedford Fenwick regarded Henry Burdett as her opponent in the battle for registration.

Ethel made a stirring and passionate speech which was recorded many years later in the *British Journal of Nursing* on 15 May 1920:

> In my opinion, Registration, to be of any value at all, must be undertaken by a legally recognised body, largely composed of the heads of the Nursing Profession themselves, with the full concurrence of medical men. We must recognise the fact that Registration is the only lever to that high, irreproachable position to which all nurses should aspire, and if unanimous, can easily attain. The time has come when this great movement is to be publicly discussed, and I call upon you ladies present, representing as you do by virtue of your office the leaders of the great army of nurses, to rise up and protect them and guard their interests with that determination and zeal which springs alone from knowledge.

The aim was to raise the standard of the profession as a whole by uniting all trained nurses, supporting and protecting their interests and providing for their registration. The stated objective was 'to unite all British nurses in membership of a recognised profession, and provide for their registration on terms satisfactory to physicians and surgeons, as evidence of their having systematic training'. To be included in the national register, nurses would have to complete their training and pass a written examination.

## Celebrations, Marriage, and New Challenges 1887–1899

An event took place in America, in Washington, on 25 March 1888, which was to eventually influence the course of Ethel Fenwick's work and the overall future of nursing. On that date, the first conference of the International Council of Women was held under the auspices of the National Women's Suffrage Association and one of the speakers, on education, was Mrs May Wright Sewell. She was eventually to become one of Ethel's great friends and an important influence in her life.

While Jack the Ripper was terrorising Whitechapel on his murderous spree between August and November 1888, development and progress continued in many different fields. Karl Benz built the first petrol-driven car. This pioneering machine had three rubber-tyred wheels and reached a speed of 9.3mph but, during a demonstration of its capabilities, Benz crashed it into a brick wall. The railway network was completed with the building of the Forth Bridge; photography became within everybody's reach with the George Eastman's invention of the Kodak camera, and the science of fingerprinting was introduced into police work.

Small changes made long-term differences in the world. The first breakfast cereal, Shredded Wheat, appeared on the market, invented by a lawyer from Colorado. The first consignment of bananas from the Canary Islands arrived in Convent Garden market in 1888 and soon regular shipments added to the variety of the British diet. In those days before paper wrappings littered the pavements, the throwing of orange-rind or peel on any footpath was amongst the many violations listed under the Street Offences Act.

George Storer, Ethel's stepfather, died in 1888 aged 73. He was buried in St Helena's churchyard at Thoroton. A portrait of his wife, Harriette, at this time revealed a tall and imposing figure with a strong nose and firm mouth wearing a widow's veil.

An important influence in the world of nursing was Princess Helena, Queen Victoria's fifth child and third daughter. Identifying herself with the nurse's cause, she became a great supporter of Ethel and her ideas. Born in 1846 as Princess Helena Augusta Victoria, she had caused concern in the royal family by becoming too fond of her father's librarian. The man was swiftly dismissed and Princess Helena was then married to HRH Prince Frederick Christian Charles Augustus of Schleswig-Holstein in 1866.

Helena, now Princess Christian, supported and worked with a number of charities including the ladies' committee of the newly founded British Red Cross, the 'Royal British Nurses' Association and the Royal School of Needlework, as well as helping to provide free school dinners for children and the unemployed in the Windsor area. Princess Christian was to prove to be a good friend and influence in Ethel's life and work; their association was long and productive. When, in 1888, Ethel gave birth to her only son, she named him Christian in honour of her friend, the Princess. As her commitment to developing a professional organisation grew, Ethel had less time to manage the Gordon House Hospital nursing home herself and eventually appointed a matron to take over her duties.

The British Nurses' Association was formally launched at public meeting in February 1888; HRH Princess Christian was approached and agreed to become the first President. A speech Princess Christian gave to a large meeting was later reported:

> The first act of the association is to obtain for the calling of nursing a recognised position and legal constitution of a profession which shall henceforth be inseparable from the noble profession of medicine. It will follow from this, that in future, every member of the nursing profession must have been educated up to a definite standard of knowledge and efficiency.

One of the early signatories, registrant number fifteen, was Ethel's friend, Anglican nun and nurse Sister Henrietta Stockdale, who became a famous nurse in South Africa and was instrumental in achieving nurse registration there in 1891 – the first country in the world to have a nurses' register.

## Celebrations, Marriage, and New Challenges 1887–1899

With the creation of the British Nurses' Association, Ethel Fenwick became the Honorary Secretary and her supportive husband became the Honorary Treasurer. Over 400 nurses and medical men joined the Association during the first few weeks, and within a year membership had reached 1,000. This was the first organisation of nurses and, from its inception, it provoked opposition from the medical profession and from hospital managers. The organisation changed its name to the Royal British Nurses' Association in 1891 and a Royal Charter was granted two years later.

The new organisation had its opponents and one of the most powerful was the organising genius, Henry Burdett. (Eventually, as Sir Henry Burdett KBC, he established the Royal National Pension Fund for Nurses and in 2002 the Burdett Trust was set up and named after this energetic philanthropist and hospital reformer.) However, having founded the Hospital Association in 1884, Burdett, as editor of its journal *The Hospital*, openly criticised the motives of founders of the British Nurses' Association. He advised readers, consisting mainly of hospital managers, to ensure that none of their nursing staff were members of the BNA.

In 1888, Henry Burdett started a section in *The Hospital* journal called 'The Nursing Mirror'. This was in response to a new and radical journal for nurses – *The Nursing Record*, 'written by nurses for nurses', which supported the BNA and the registration cause. Ethel was implacably hostile towards Henry Burdett, blaming him for the delay in registration, although initially Florence Nightingale was a far more effective opponent.

Registration was passionately debated throughout the 1880s and 1890s. Florence Nightingale employed her formidable talents and influence in the registration battle but she was not fundamentally opposed to the idea of registry. Many hospitals kept their own records but, believing it to be purely a vocational calling, Florence objected to the idea that nursing was simply a 'profession', and used that word in a pejorative sense.

Unlike the BNA, which wanted to raise the social status of nursing and exclude the less well educated, Florence Nightingale strongly believed that lack of a formal education should not preclude a woman from becoming a good nurse and she advocated improving the general quality of nursing care by improved training. She also objected to the registry because of the problems of keeping it accurate and updated. No mechanism existed for removing names of nurses deemed subsequently unfit, which meant the register was inaccurate. Also, the proposed register did not list where a nurse received her training or if she had received any additional training – as training programmes varied considerably in quality this meant information on the register was a virtually useless means of assessing a nurse's capabilities.

Matrons of nursing homes feared that, once they were unable to take in probationers for 'training', their wages bill would soar. Although it was first mooted in Great Britain, nurses achieved registration in many other countries before the Registration Act was finally passed in Britain. Later, controversial modern historian Professor Abel-Smith wrote in 1960, describing the battle for registration 'as a battle for status conducted against a background of rampant snobbery and militant feminism'. The British Medical Association was consistently in favour of registration but, with money being a great concern, many individual doctors disagreed. One wrote in the *Nursing Record* of January 1897 that 'this new profession is taking a very large sum that would otherwise go to the doctors, represented by many thousands of pounds'. These contentious views give an insight into the strength of feeling aroused during those fractious early days.

The nurses' registration debate grew intense, eventually even impinging on the public consciousness, but the BNA had a great social advantage in having Princess Christian as their President. Her presence inhibited more severe criticism and turned meetings into dazzling affairs. Florence Nightingale objected strongly to the granting of a Royal Charter to the BNA in 1889.

In 1889, a group of people, including Dr Bedford Fenwick, had petitioned for a Select Committee to examine the conditions under which nurses worked at the London Hospital. An old rivalry for the affections of Dr Bedford Fenwick had resulted in uncompromising animosity between Matron Eva Luckes and Ethel, which undoubtedly coloured their attitudes towards each other. As a result of the petition, the Select Committee of the House of Lords on Metropolitan Hospitals met between 1890 and 1892. The *Nursing Record* reported weekly on the evidence put before the committee, and included highly critical comments about Miss Eva Luckes – 'The London nurses worked in circumstances of danger, hardship, overwork and bad housing and their vocational spirit was exploited.' At the London Hospital, nurses were expected to work from 7.00 am–9.00 pm with half an hour for lunch. Pay was £10 a year.

In the 1890s, there were hardly any male nurses and no London hospital would accept them for training. A Mr Michael Walsh ran the Male Nurses' Temperance Cooperation in London and was of the opinion that those who had previously been gentlemen's servants made the best nurses. Men of higher social status were not deemed able to manage violent patients, and 'invitations to dinner and boxes at the theatre were apt to interfere with their professional engagements'. (Numbers of male nurses increased very slowly – by 1937 only 120 were in training.)

In 1894, in *Women's Work*, A. Bulley and M. Whitely wrote:

> a good deal of mischief arises from the mistaken notions as to what the profession of nursing ought to be. Nurses are supposed to take it up in missionary spirit for the good of the community, without regard to their own comfort and health. Now unfortunately, the more 'noble' a profession is considered, the greater is the tendency to neglect the material well-being of those concerned in it.

While the large hospitals were staffed by trained nurses, and able to attract the best recruits, smaller hospitals had to make do with a lower calibre of entrants. The destitute sick could be nursed in asylums, but many people were nursed in their own homes. The upper and middle classes would often employ women who called themselves 'hospital-trained', many of whom had failed to complete their training and were anxious to earn more money as private nurses. Some were willing to describe themselves as 'certified' without any hospital experience, and some doctors were willing to give 'certificates' to any nurse who had worked for them.

The insane were kept in large asylums well away from towns, 'out of sight and out of mind'. Psychiatric care was mainly custodial, within asylums, and any 'cures' that occurred were due to spontaneous recovery from mental illness. The Medical Psychological Association had been founded in 1841 and later obtained a Royal Charter. It had published a handbook on mental nursing in 1885, started a three-year training scheme and began to issue certificates. Recruits for this specialist training were few, but eventually a special register for mental nurses was established in 1919.

The Infectious Diseases (Notification) Act of 1889 gives an insight into medical problems of the day and lists 'smallpox, cholera, diphtheria fever, membranous croup, erysipelas, scarlatina or scarlet fever, and the fevers known as typhus, typhoid, enteric, relapsing continued, or puerperal and any other scheduled by a Local Authority' as diseases that must be notified to the Medical Officer of Health of the district. A daunting list of fines were imposed for failing to comply with regulations for disposing of infected material and exposing or conveying infected persons, disinfecting clothing, bedding and articles used by an infected person.

The world of nursing was not the only area requiring change in this time. By 1888, political and social reformer Keir Hardie had helped to form the Scottish Parliamentary Fabian Party and many reformers were highlighting cases of exploitation. Typical of these was Annie Bessant, journalist, theosophist, and early champion of contraception, who wrote a chilling account when campaigning for London match-workers. She described how the huge profits that the shareholders enjoyed were actually made from the labour of young girls working in appallingly dangerous and exhausting conditions. She gave the example of one girl who, at the cost of damaging a machine, had been fined for trying to prevent the loss of her fingers. Ignoring such problems, and determined to show his admiration for Mr Gladstone, the owner of the factory, Theodore Bryant, had decided to erect a statue to the great man and 'allowed his workers to contribute' by stopping money out of their wages. Annie Bessant's explicit article caused tremendous outrage, leading to a boycott and eventually a factory strike.

An old police manual gives an insight into transport of the time when, in the Police Offences Act of 1892 relating to street offences, the term carriage is defined as 'any coach, omnibus, tram-way car cab, cabriolet, gig, brougham, wagon, timber-carriage, dray, truck, cart, hand-cart, wheelbarrow, lorry, bicycle, tricycle, velocipede'.

In 1890, the last major conflict between Native Americans and United States troops took place at Wounded Knee, South Dakota. Also in America, the innovative surgeon William S. Halstead (1852–1922) began the use of sterile rubber gloves in the operating theatre, thereby drastically reducing the incidences of infection.

The cause of Irish Independence was put at risk and set back many years when the love affair between Irish leader Charles Parnell and married woman Kitty O'Shea was made public. In 1892, Keir Hardie was elected as Member of Parliament for West Ham, and helped in the formation of the independent Labour party.

Ethel Fenwick remained interested in antiques and continued to indulge her appreciation of fine tastes and quality. She was always very fashion-conscious as this description of her attending a function in 1890 illustrates: 'wearing a most artistic dress of apple green satin draped with black net, exquisitely embroidered with white lilies and green jeweled leaves and a long black velvet train; she wore only one jewel, a beautiful diamond and emerald heart, and the Order of St. John of Jerusalem'. Ethel's husband was by now a distinguished specialist in Wimpole Street, Ethel was busy with her campaign and so, as was the convention of the time, their reliable nanny dedicated herself to the care of their young son, Christian. The growing child spent a lot of the time in the healthier environment of Dunningwell, home of Ethel's sister, Clara.

Opposition to registration of nurses was largely based on tenuous moral grounds. Matron of the London Hospital, Eva Luckes, and her mentor Florence Nightingale were vigorously opposed to registration, believing that the essential moral qualities that made a good nurse would be subordinate to theories and exams. A friend of Florence Nightingale, Sir Henry Bonham-Carter, concluded in a pamphlet that 'registration was not desirable since moral as well as professional qualities are everything in a nurse, and these cannot be measured, or kept up to date in a record'. Florence Nightingale was indignant at the support given to the BNA by eminent doctors who, she believed, knew nothing at all about such matters as nurse training. When Sir James Paget asked why nurses couldn't lodge out as other students did at the time, Miss Nightingale was horrified at the suggestion, believing it illustrated his ignorance on the vocational aspect of nursing.

Meantime, throughout all the battles, Ethel had not confined herself to a single field of operations. She was appointed a member of the Women's Committee of the British Royal Commission for the World's Fair opening in Chicago in May 1893 and was invited to superintend the exhibition of nursing effects. She had a germ of another inspirational idea and wrote in the *Nursing Record* of 6 October 1892:

> I am going next week to America as the delegate of the Royal Commission to arrange about the exhibits of British Women's work … I shall try to persuade our Nursing Sisters to arrange for an International Nursing Congress to meet during the Exhibition. It would be the first Congress of the kind which I believe has ever been held.

Ethel crossed the Atlantic, taking around a week to do so, on one of the White Star Line ships in October 1892. She went to make arrangements for the exhibition and planned: 'On two inlaid pedestals will stand

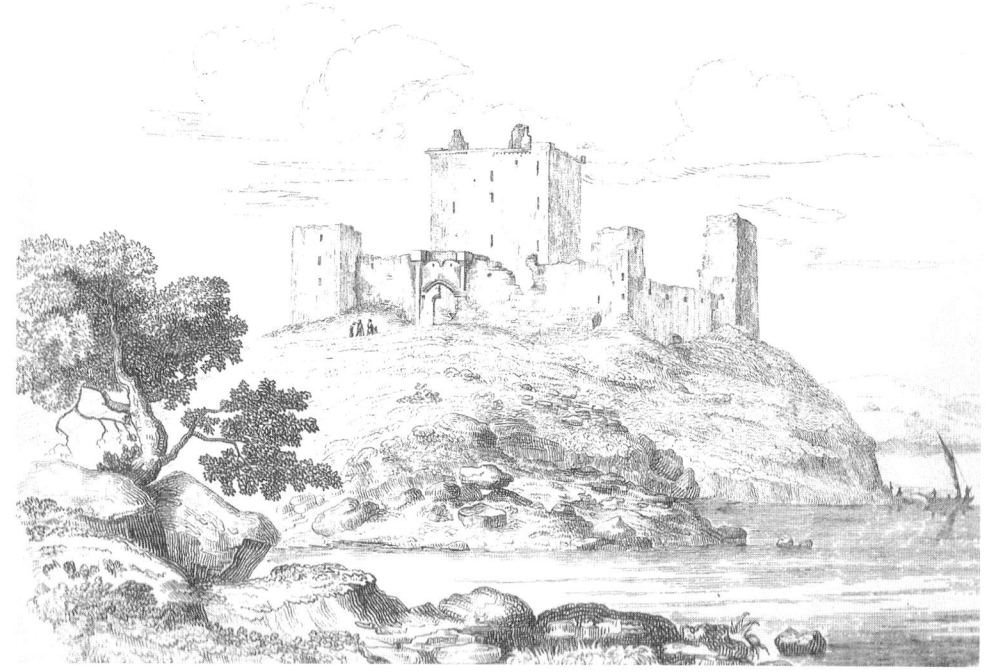

Spynie Palace ruins in 1839. (*J. Main*)

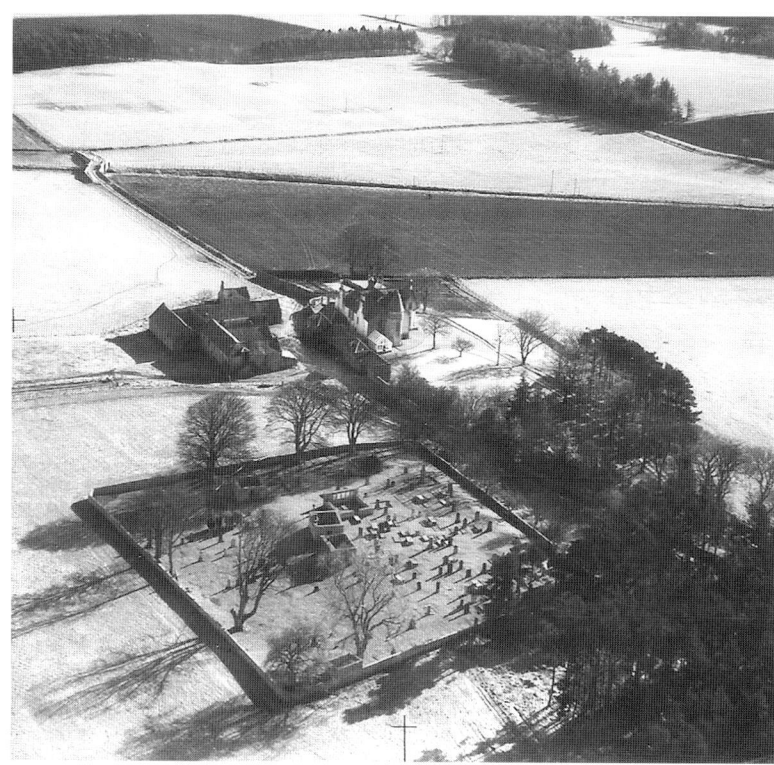

Aerial view of Spynie House and Churchyard, c.1970. (*J. Main*)

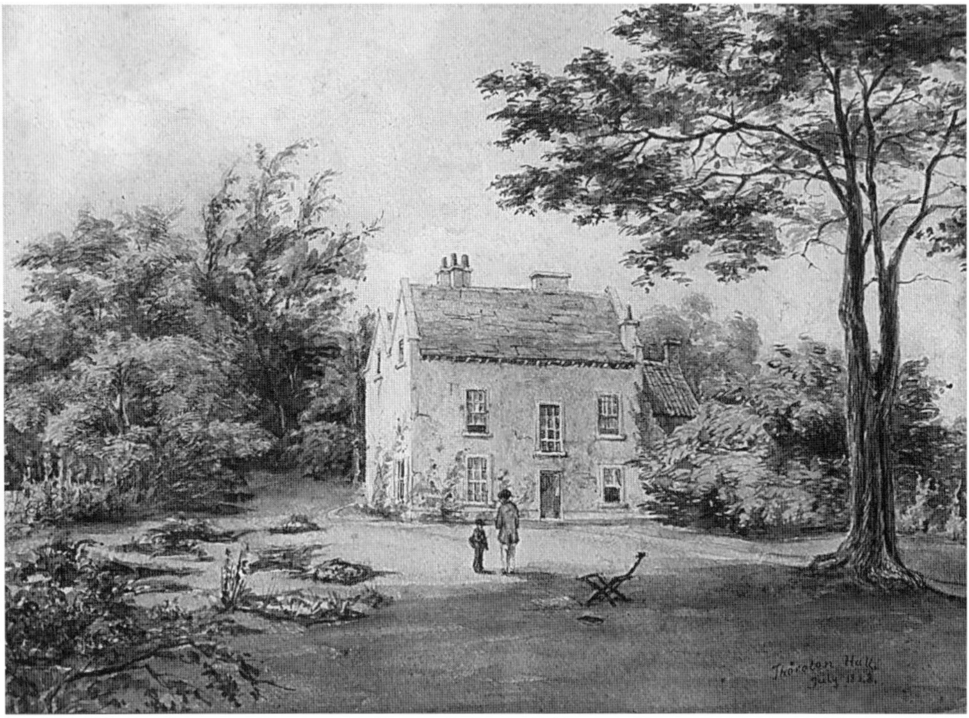

Thoroton Hall c.1860s (*J. O'Reilly*)

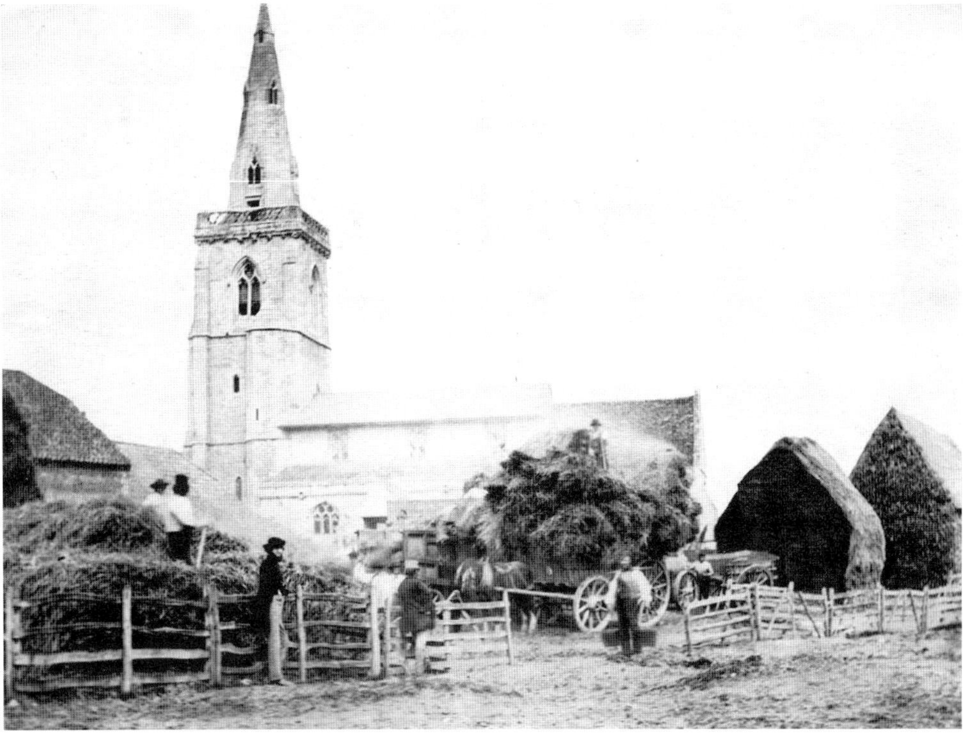

Thoroton Church, late 1800s. (*Catherine Clarke*)

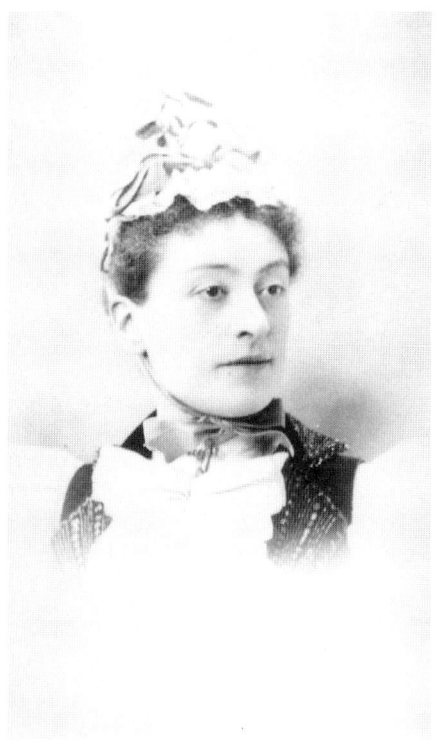

The young nurse – Ethel Gordon Manson. (*Archives, St Bartholomew's*)

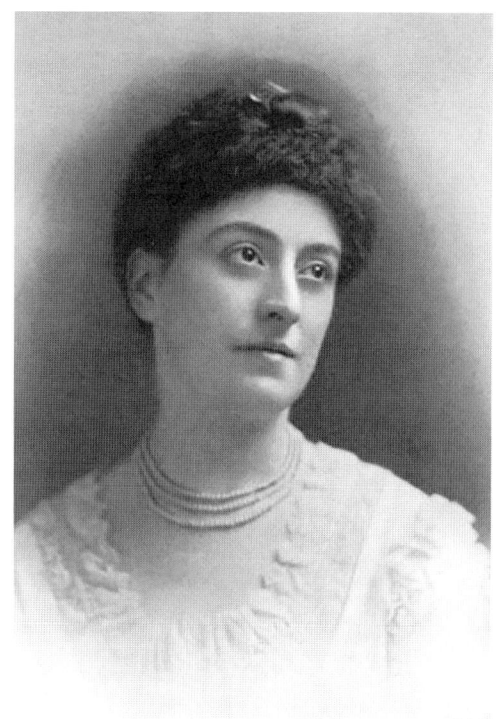

Ethel Gordon Manson. (*Archives, St Bartholomew's*)

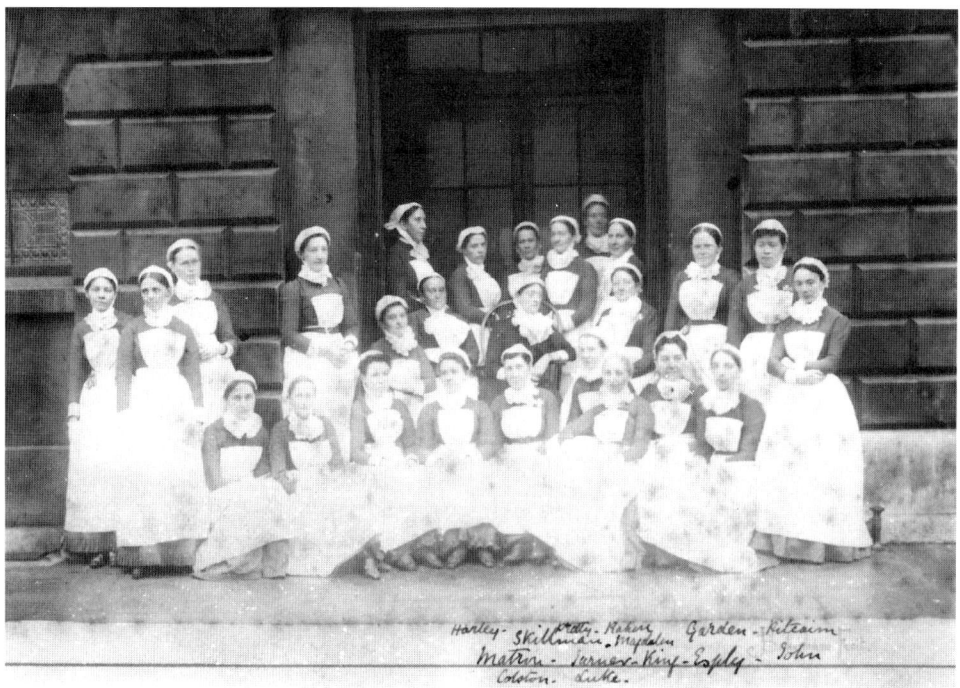

Ethel Manson, Matron, with her nurses at St Bartholomew's. (*Archives, St Bartholomew's*)

St Bartholomew's nurse with coal scuttle, c.1890. (*Wellcome Images*)

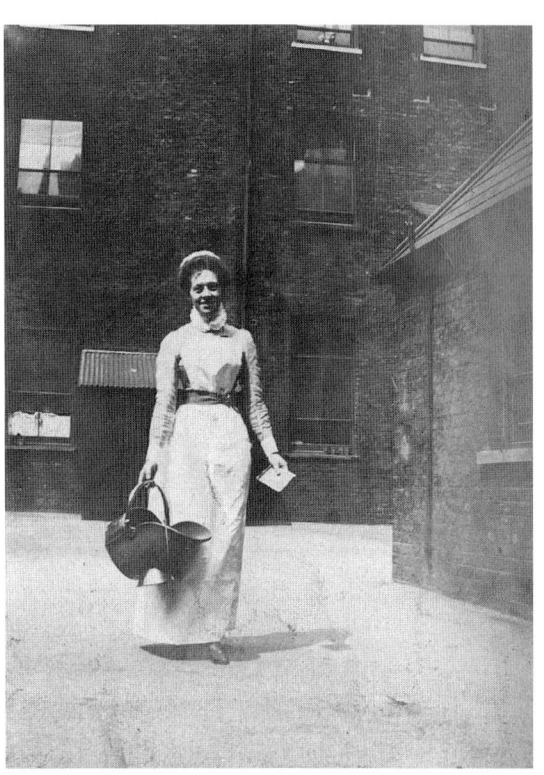

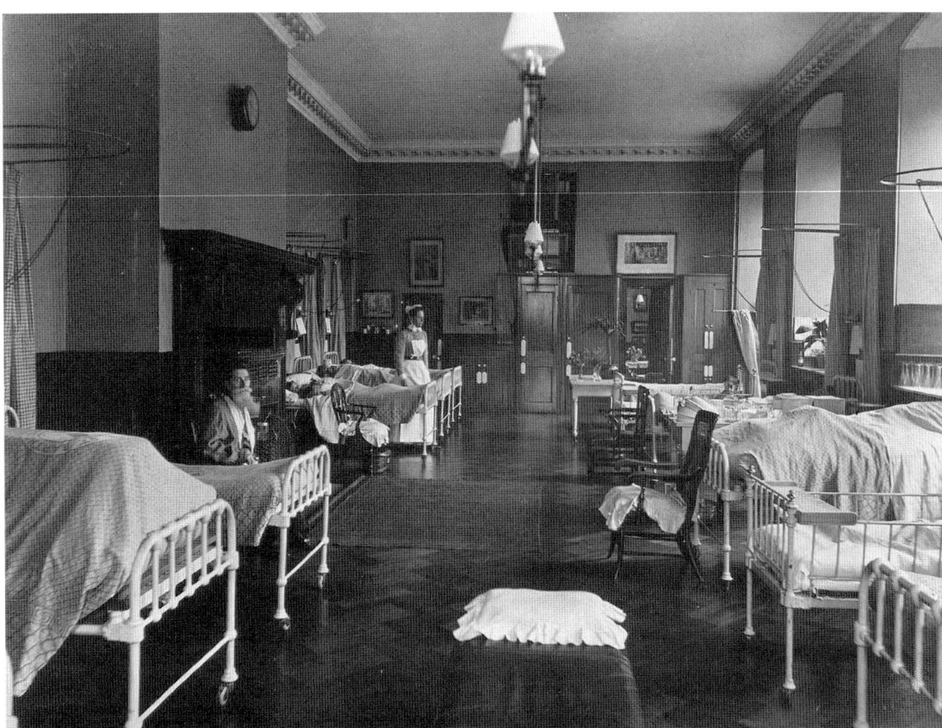

St Bartholomew's hospital ward, c.1890. (*Wellcome Images*)

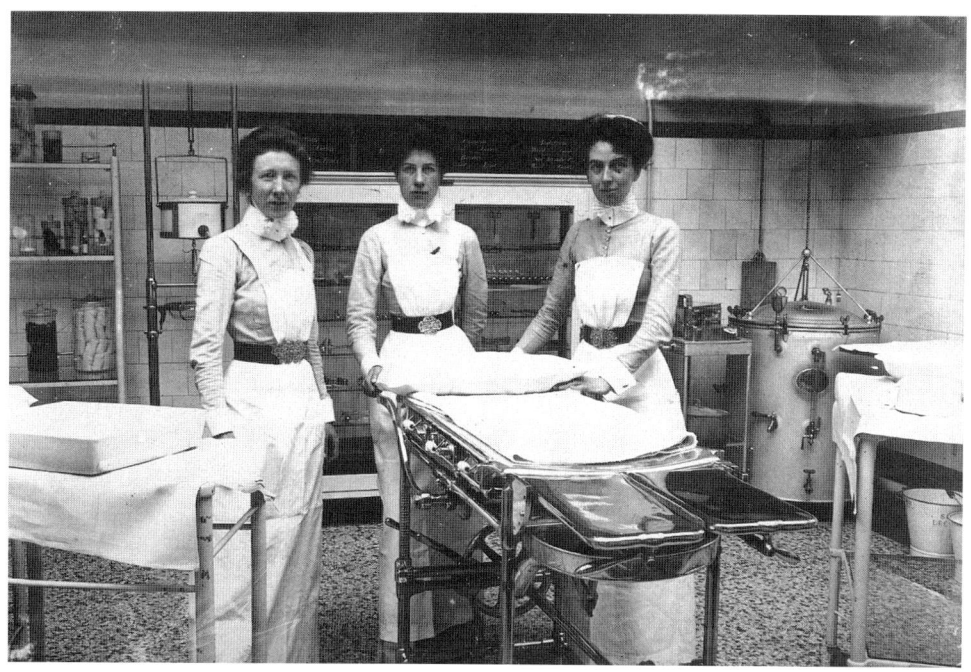

St Bartholomew's operating theatre, c.1890. (*Wellcome Images*)

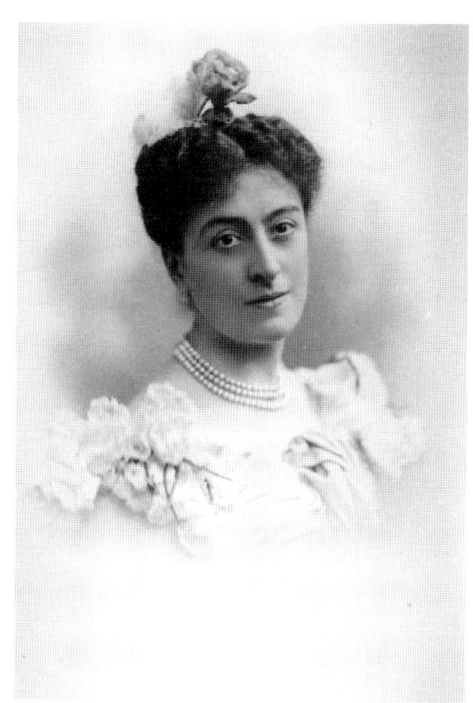

Mrs Ethel Bedford Fenwick in her finery. (*Archives, St Bartholomew's*)

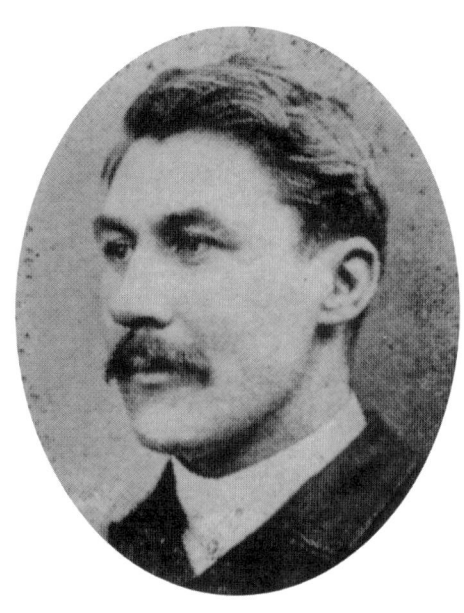

Dr Bedford Fenwick. (*Archives, St Bartholomew's*)

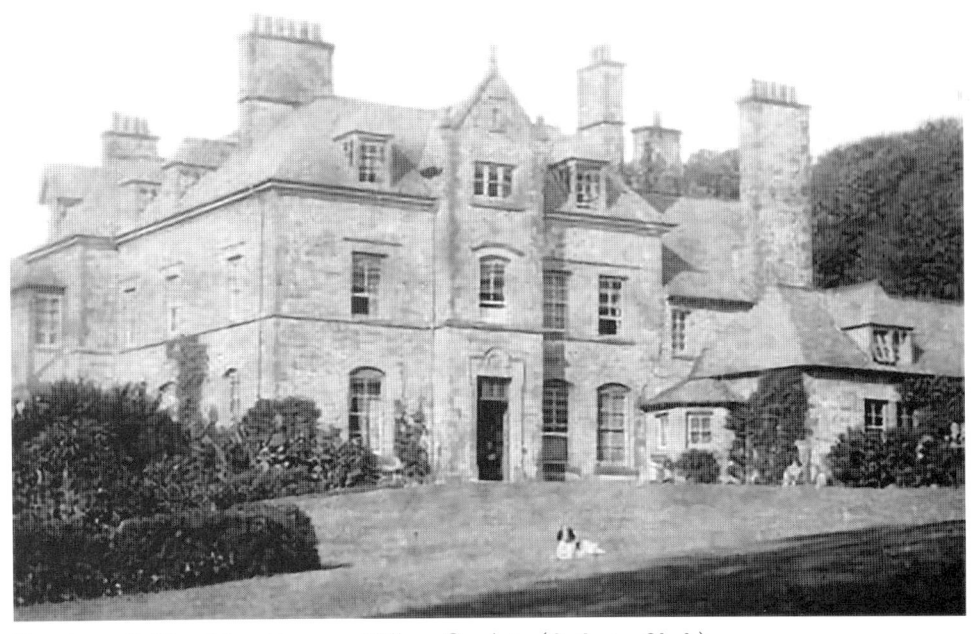

Dunningwell, Clara Myers' home at Millom, Cumbria. (*Catherine Clarke*)

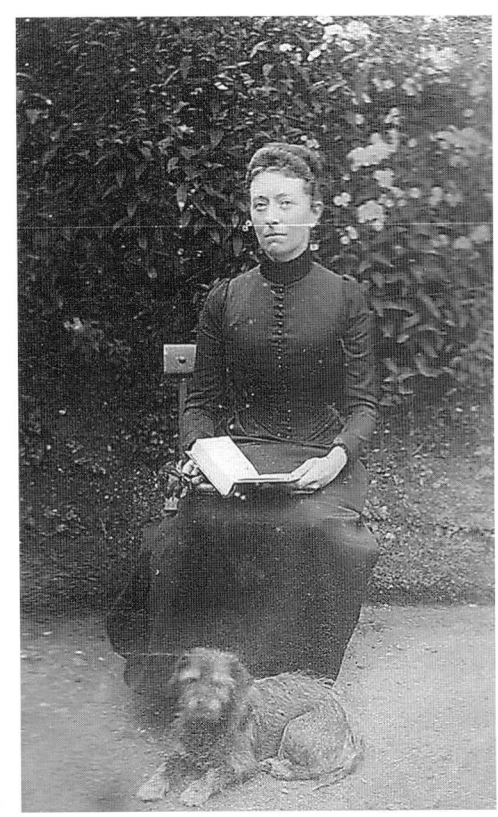

Ethel's sister Clara Myers. (*Catherine Clarke*)

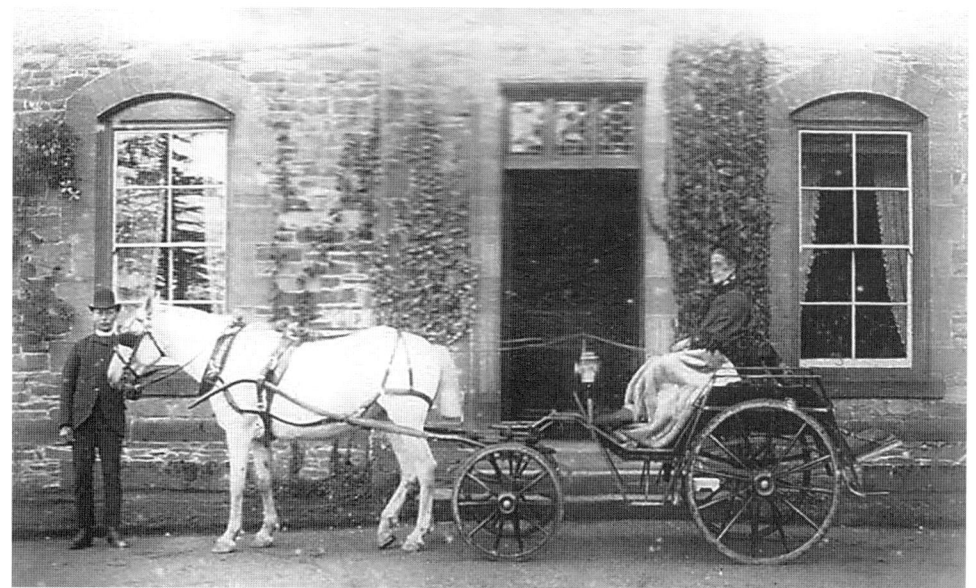

Clara Myers in her carriage at Dunningwell. (*Catherine Clarke*)

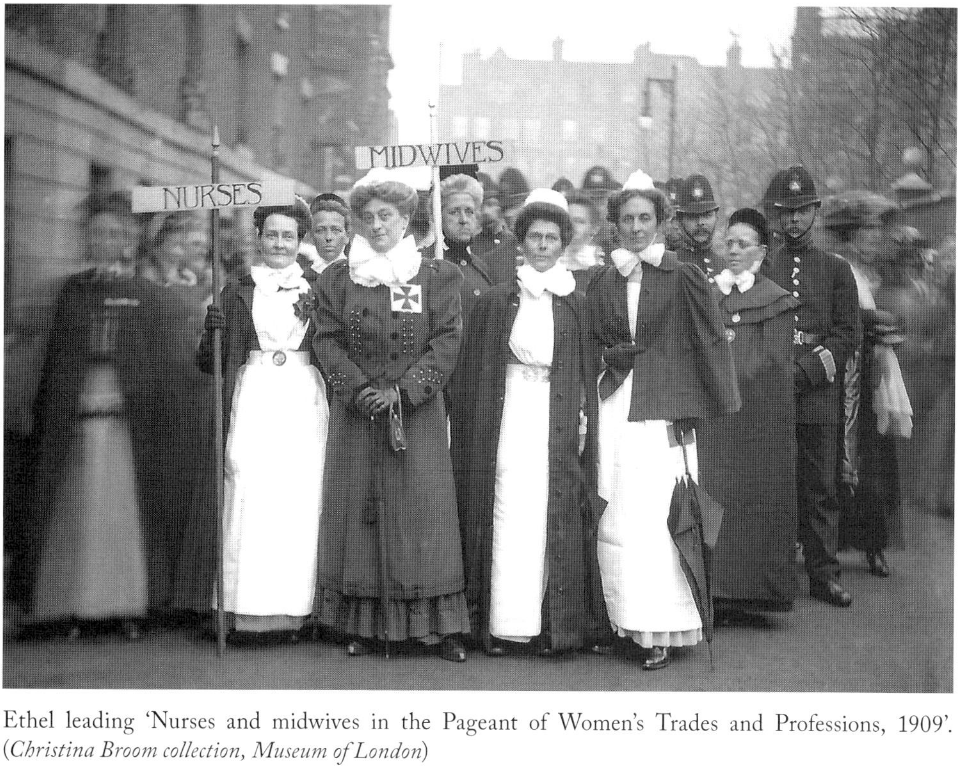

Ethel leading 'Nurses and midwives in the Pageant of Women's Trades and Professions, 1909'. (*Christina Broom collection, Museum of London*)

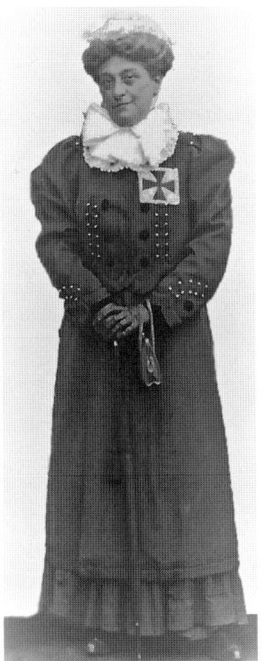

Ethel Gordon Fenwick. (*Archives, St Bartholomew's*)

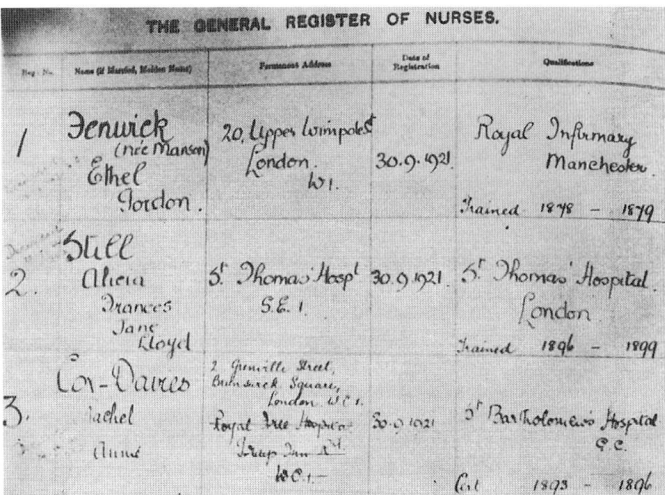

The first signature. (*Winifred Hector*)

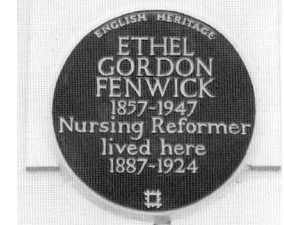

The Blue Plaque outside Ethel's Wimpole Street home. (*J. Main*)

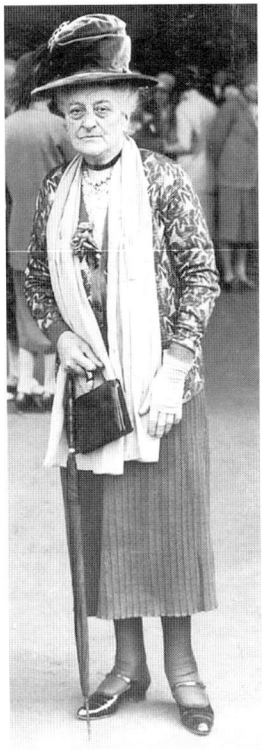

The older Ethel Gordon Fenwick. (*Archives, St Bartholomew's*)

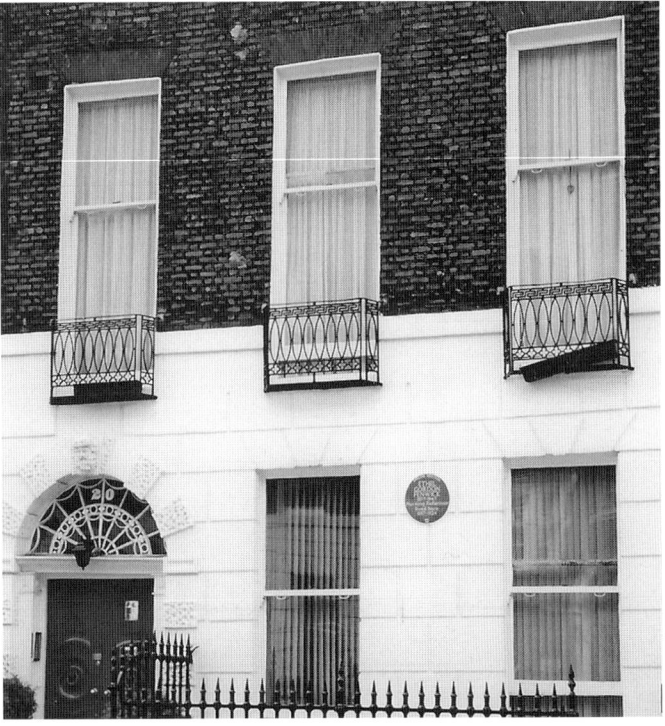

Ethel's home in Wimpole Street, c.2000. (*J. Main*)

the bust of our President (Mrs. Fenwick) and Rahere, the founder of St. Bartholomew's, our oldest and most famous hospital and training school.'

The British Nursing section of the exhibition contained every kind of appliance, bandages, and operation gowns. Toothbrushes were made from ox bone and bristle. (Bone brush production was eventually discontinued in 1947.) In a centre glass case were sixty dolls, 17 inches high, in uniform. There was a beautiful picture of the Queen and an inlaid bookcase with a complete nursing library. One exhibit was the 'ward toilet basket' – a brown plate basket divided in the middle and lined with red American cloth, 'with loose cover of the same, on the one side fits a boxwood Plasmon powder box and a covered glass bottle for rectified spirits, brush and comb, nailbrush, small tooth comb, scissors and soap-case; on the other side is a dusting brush, whisk brush for mattresses, dusters, and a bottle of Sharps metal polish'. For her efforts, Ethel received two medals of distinction.

Ethel Fenwick crossed the Atlantic again, in April 1893, to attend the Congress of Representative Women held in Chicago during the World Fair. This was to prove a most fruitful expedition, where meeting with several influential women helped her to formulate new ideas and plans of action. Her expertise and authority were recognised and much respected and, while in America, she was treated as an honoured guest and was taken to visit some of the technically more advanced major training hospitals. She found steam sterilisation of dressings in general use, and sterile packs stored in airtight jars.

During her visit to Johns Hopkins Hospital in Baltimore, Ethel met Lavinia Dock, assistant director of the nursing department. Their meeting was one of major importance as they soon discovered themselves to be kindred spirits and became lifelong friends. Lavinia was a distinguished nurse and authoress, and an ardent supporter of women's suffrage. Both women firmly believed, in Ethel Fenwick's words – 'the nurse's question was the women's question'.

Miss Dock had written:

to attain such an end (professional organisation) where women are concerned arouses prehistoric prejudices and touches a multitude of vested interests. Hence the stringent opposition with which every effort of nursing reform has been and is being met ... the industrial spinster does not count, she is a voteless item of humanity.

(*American Journal of Nursing*, 1901)

Ethel's ideas on the status of nurses were strongly influenced by her contact with the American nurses. As well as the ardent feminist and nursing director, Lavinia Dock, Ethel Fenwick came in contact with two leading nurse educationalists, Adelaide Nutting and Annie Goodrich. Impressed by advances in America where some hospitals had adopted the non-payment of probationers and treated them as pupils, Ethel Fenwick advocated the 'collegiate' system, with pupils paying for cost of training, partly in money and partly in labour. In 1895 she was writing that the English system of nurse training was unsatisfactory due to the probationers' training being secondary to the manpower needs of the hospital. This was a debate that was to continue for very many years.

During the 1893 trip to the Chicago Fair, Ethel also became involved with the International Council of Women, following a meeting with another determined woman, Mrs May Wright Sewell, founder of the ICW. The two formed a strong friendship and their meeting was to set the seeds of another new enterprise. The first conference of the ICW had been held in Washington, on 25 March 1888, under the auspices of the National Women's Suffrage Association. Ethel was determined to try to persuade the Nursing Sisters to arrange for an International Nursing Congress. Although this did not materialise immediately, she remained determined to achieve this worldwide Nursing Congress. The final impetus for its creation was to come some years later during the next International Council of Women, held in London in 1899.

Back in Britain, having been granted the prefix 'Royal', the British Nursing Association applied for a Royal Charter of incorporation. The application was strongly resisted by all opponents of registration who feared this would make the Royal BNA too powerful and that its influence would be a threat to the medical authorities and the smooth running of hospitals. In the pages of the *Nursing Record* and *The Hospital*, Mrs Fenwick and Mr Burdett accused each other of unworthy motives. To her, he represented the vested interest of employers and male arrogance. To him, the RBNA represented the cutting edge of organised labour and women's rights. A Privy Council inquiry was held, which eventually decided in favour of granting a charter in 1893.

Ethel Fenwick was jubilant. This was the first occasion that a Royal Charter had been granted to an association of professional women and she saw it as the recognition of the RBNA as a professional body. However, it was a pyrrhic victory. The powers granted were not so extensive as those which had been sought, and the byelaws had been subtly altered. The power to maintain a register of nurses had been applied for, but only the power to maintain a list of nurses was granted. No rights or privileges were given to the members of the Chartered Corporation, nor had any nurse the right to call herself chartered or registered. Even so, this was some small improvement on the voluntary register, which the association had started in 1891. The tide was turning and now Florence Nightingale admitted that, on the subject of registration, 'Forty years hence, such a scheme might not be preposterous', and she took no further active part in the controversy.

Always perceptive and aware of the power of publicity, Dr and Mrs Fenwick took over the *Nursing Record* in 1893 (to become the *British Journal of Nursing* in 1902), with Ethel becoming the honorary editor. Both had previously contributed articles to the journal, he on medical nursing, she on education and the organisation of nurses. She began to encourage nurses to study their patients and conditions more closely and to make a 'case history' for which prizes of books were awarded. In her first editorial, Mrs Fenwick announced that the goal of the *Nursing Record* was to accomplish state registration for nurses. The battle for registration was becoming fiercer and the weapon of publicity was wielded with determination. By 1894, she began including a column called 'Women', which reported on suffragist meetings, women's union affairs, and news of all feminine organisations. Her articles were in direct opposition to those of Henry Burnet, who was writing in 'The Nursing Mirror', a section of *The Hospital* journal.

In 1894, a correspondent in the *Nursing Times* observed that, while adequate financial and social rewards were open to men who were prepared to work well, few women, unless prepared to go on the stage, could earn more than the barest living. She then declared that women would always be helpless and despised until they had power to make money and had a voice in the making of the laws. Meanwhile, in New Zealand, women had managed to obtain the vote by 1893.

As the campaign for registration lengthened into decades, and opposing sides became more entrenched, Ethel Fenwick's pen never spared her opponents, despite one of them being from Ethel's old hospital. Eva Luckes, Matron of the London Hospital, had written a pamphlet questioning the need for an association of nurses and the value of registration. The battle for registration went far beyond the old rivalries and passionate personality clashes between these two arch enemies.

Not surprisingly amongst a group of such opinionated people, strife broke out within the ranks of the RBNA and, following a change in the regulations instigated by their opponents, the Bedford Fenwicks lost office. At a joint meeting between the BMA and nurses' representatives to discuss registration, the RBNA delegates voted for a resolution which stated that state registration 'was inexpedient in principle, injurious to the best interest of nurses, and of doubtful public benefit'.

In 1894, thinking that a group of these powerful women would undoubtedly help further the cause of registration, Ethel founded the Matrons' Council, along with her close friend and successor as Matron of St Bartholomew's, Isla Stewart. In 1896, Ethel Fenwick organised a major nursing exhibition and conference to promote 'scientific nursing'. The aim was to provide nurses with the opportunity to see the latest appliances and inventions for nursing the sick. She hoped to raise professional awareness by eliciting opinions of nurses on subjects, including registration, and to demonstrate to the public the determination of nurses. She contributed a paper on 'nursing of our soldiers'. The whole venture was a definite success and Ethel realised that the forthcoming Congress of the International Council of Women, to be held in London in 1899, would be the perfect opportunity to hold an international conference for nurses. Her dream of an International Congress of Nurses seemed to be nearing realisation.

By 1897, Mr Burdett had become President of the RBNA and in 1899, the voluntary registration of nurses was replaced by the simple membership roll of the Association. Ethel had to look elsewhere for support for professional registration on the journey to reform that would prove to be unexpectedly long, difficult, and highly contentious.

The year 1897 saw the outbreak of the Graeco-Turkish War and, when Ethel Fenwick was appointed Secretary of the National Fund for Crete, she set about organising a group of British nurses to assist the Greeks. When it seemed that the hospitals were not coping very well, she set out personally to organise them, believing she must do it herself because, as she said, 'it would certainly be difficult and possibly dangerous'. The dispatches she sent back for her magazine were reminiscent of those of a war correspondent, and certainly provided lively copy.

It was a complicated issue – European powers became embroiled in the Graeco-Turkish squabble – which was a precursor of troubles soon to come. This first Graeco-Turkish War, also called the Thirty Days' War, took place against a background of growing Greek concern over conditions in Crete, under Turkish domination and where relations between Christians and their Muslim rulers had been deteriorating. The outbreak in 1896 of rebellion in Crete, fomented in part by the secret Greek nationalist society, appeared to present Greece with an opportunity to annex the island. By 1897, large consignments of arms had been sent to Crete from Greece. In January, the Greek fleet was mobilised and in February, Greek troops landed on the island and union with Greece was proclaimed. By the following month, in order to prevent the disturbance spreading to the Balkans, European powers became involved. After much fighting and European pressure, the Greeks withdrew their troops from Crete. Turkish troops also left Crete, which had been made an international protectorate, and a peace treaty was concluded in December. Crete was finally ceded to Greece by the Treaty of London in 1913, which ended the first Balkan War.

The National Fund for the Greek Wounded had been started by the *Daily Chronicle* in order to send nurses and supplies to Greece during the Graeco-Turkish War. The first twenty nurses were selected by Ethel Fenwick and they went out to Greece in April 1897. Not content with simple organisation, she went to Athens in May and took over as superintendent of nursing in military hospitals. Her impressive hard work was admired, particularly by Queen Olga of the Hellenes and her daughter-in-law, Crown Princess Sophie, who often visited the Ecole Militaire Hospital. In recognition of her efforts, Ethel Fenwick was later awarded the Distinguished Order and the Diploma of the Greek Red Cross.

Never one to rest on her laurels, on her return to Britain Ethel plunged back into the fray, helping to promote the work of the International Council of Women for their forthcoming Congress. She was appointed a member of the committee to arrange the programme for the future Congress to be held in London in 1899.

Around this time, an unheralded but life-changing advance in medicine occurred when aspirin was developed by a German chemist, Felix Hoffmann, who was searching for a treatment for his father's arthritis. The basic ingredients had been known as long ago as the fifth century BC, when Hippocrates is reputed to have used ground willow bark (which contains salicin) to ease aches and pains. Research by Thomas Maclagan in Dundee during the 1860s had led to the development and use of salicylates but Hoffman managed to create a drug that was less harsh or irritating to the stomach.

By 1897, it was apparent that the fight for women's suffrage would be a difficult one, and in order to achieve a more effective and coherent organisation, the various suffragist societies united into one National Union of Women's Suffrage Societies. However, one group, impatient and frustrated at government inaction, became more militant under the leadership of Emmeline Pankhurst and her daughter Christabel.

The year 1897 marked Queen Victoria's Diamond Jubilee and the banquet at Buckingham Palace on the eve of the Jubilee was the first occasion in her widowhood that Victoria did not wear black. This Jubilee was celebrated with an enormous procession, during which the Prince of Wales rode on one side of his elderly mother's carriage, his cousin the Kaiser on the other, escorted by 50,000 troops. Queen Victoria was dressed in grey and black, with a black lace parasol trimmed with white. There was much flag waving, several large garden parties, and many grand society dinners and balls. Imperialism was the dominant creed; the Crown was the symbol of British Imperialism with the Queen representing the ideals and achievements of the Great British Empire – self-perceived as superior and invincible.

Some spectators of the mighty procession were not entirely impressed. The artist Edward Burne-Jones recorded his observations:

> It was all surprisingly successful – but all the boasting of the papers is so dreadful; it makes one wonder that a thunderbolt doesn't fall upon London. They're so silly as not to know that the gods do not love the pride of cockiness. There was one set of men near where we were, that won great favour. It was a regiment that kept the ground in front of Downing Street – the Seaforth Highlanders. They were in the highest good humour with everybody, and the pipers puffed away and kept walking backwards and forwards swelling with such pride and excitement that their naked calves seemed to turn upwards – making such a beastly row that I loathe and detest above all others – till I nearly went mad. Excellent people no doubt and in the best of tempers they were, but in that dress with tight plaid trousers and huge head-dress of ostrich feathers they looked like South Sea Islanders altogether. There was an old boy on horseback

who kept riding up and down and screaming at them and you could see his ridiculous bottom as he sat on his saddle. And he had brass-coloured eyebrows and moustaches and a pink face.

At a Jubilee garden party at Buckingham Palace, Queen Victoria was escorted by great numbers of Indian cavalry officers, men in handsome uniforms and great boots. She sat in a large tent banked up with flowers and open at the front so that her faithful subjects could see her taking tea and having her toast buttered by her Indian servant. One of the large marquees was not open and the heat became stifling. Lord Esher was present in his court dress and used his rapier to cut openings in the canvas – until stopped by a yell from a royal housemaid, whom he had inadvertently stabbed.

Amongst the many great parties, the grandest was given by the Duchess of Devonshire, who held a fancy-dress ball which all the aristocracy, including the Prince and Princess of Wales, attended. Herbert Asquith went as a roundhead soldier and his wife as a snake charmer. The new Poet Laureate wrote a dreadful Jubilee poem, as did Francis Thompson, whose offering began 'Night, and the street a corpse beneath the moon'.

Rudyard Kipling redeemed the situation with his famous 'Recessional', the chorus of 'Lest we forget' and the last lines giving a warning: 'For frantic boast and foolish word – Thy mercy on Thy People Lord.'

Around this time, Kipling wrote percipiently to a friend about his fears for the future: 'The big smash is coming one of these days, sure enough, but I think we shall pull through … It will be the common people – the third-class carriages – that'll save us.' Kipling was overjoyed a few months later at the birth of his son John – but the 'big smash' did come when Britain went to war against Germany and his beloved John, by then a subaltern in the Irish Guards, was one of the millions of casualties. But that lay in the future, and in 1887 the Kaiser and the Prince of Wales together escorted Queen Victoria through her Jubilee parade in an ostentatious display of harmony.

# Celebrations, Marriage, and New Challenges 1887–1899

Another who sensed trouble ahead, Field Marshal Lord Wolsey, was stirred by reports of some upper-class excess, and wrote to his wife these prophetic words:

> I feel that a country whose upper classes live as a certain set of men and women do, can only be saved from annihilation by some such upheaval as a great war, which will cost all the best families their sons, and call forth both the worst animal passions and the noblest of human virtues, and for the time place the very existence of the kingdom in danger.

Some enterprising adventurers managed to break out of the unequal social system by emigrating. When, in 1896, gold was discovered at Bonanza Creek in Klondike, 60,000 prospectors flooded in, and by 1900, £30 million had been mined. Dawson burgeoned from a small mining camp into a town of 20,000 settlers.

In Britain, the book *Child of the Jago*, published by journalist Arthur Morrison, revealed horrendous insights into the life of the poor in London's East End and became a publishing sensation. Life was also hard for the rural poor, who considered it normal to have to walk many miles daily to get to and from work, and whose sufferings were not often considered by their employers. There was little doubt that the Victorian world consisted of pre-ordained classes and class distinction was a fact of life. Queen Victoria and other establishment figures were unaware of the true squalor and suffering of the poor. While she took great interest in the 'crofters' around her estate at Balmoral, the Queen remained ignorant of the conditions of rural poverty and any protests were perceived to be threats of revolutionaries, menacing the stable order of society and of government. However, changes in the agricultural scene were heralding a slow end to the accustomed order, and positions such as those of footmen, grooms and other servants were gradually disappearing.

In Dundee, Dr George Alexander Pirie persisted doggedly at his pioneering development of X-rays. His determination and devotion to continue working with such a dangerous and uncontrolled new substance led eventually to the amputation of both his hands, loss of his eyesight and finally resulted in his death. In America, in 1896, the first X-ray photograph was made by Dr Henry Louis Smith, who fired a bullet into a corpse. He then took and developed an X-ray exposure which showed the exact location of the bullet. Working quietly but persistently, the remarkable Marie Curie discovered radioactivity in 1898 and the world of medicine began to change inexorably. The British Empire was plunged into turmoil with the beginning, in 1899, of the Boer War, which was to prove the most expensive of British Imperial exploits and the beginning of the long decline of Empire.

Concentrating on issues at home in 1899, Keir Hardie, now the Labour leader, savaged Lord Overtoun, the owner of a huge chemical works in Rutherglen. Lord Overtoun lived in a magnificent Dumbarton mansion, was a pillar of the Free Church and had campaigned against the opening of the People's Palace on the Sabbath. The People's Palace on Glasgow Green had been built in the most deprived area of Glasgow and was intended as a cultural centre and a meeting place for the local people. It was opened in 1898 by the Earl of Roseberry, who stated that it would be 'a Palace of pleasure and imagination around which people may place their affections and which may give them a home on which their memory may rest', before declaring it 'open to the people for ever and ever'.

However, Lord Overtoun objected to any Sunday opening on religious grounds – while at the same time requiring his own people to work twelve hours a day, seven days a week, without a single meal break. He was a philanthropist who contributed three guineas a year to the Glasgow Hospital for Skin Diseases while, at his Shawfields works in Rutherglen, men were being casually poisoned by the black liquid dripping on their skin.

Enraged by these double standards and by the conditions at the Shawfield works, Keir Hardie exposed the realities of the situation by writing:

If the men had a scratch, the poison slowly burns its festering way through their flesh until the bone is reached, and then the putrid flesh drops out, leaving a hole so large that a man's thumb won't cover it ... In some case it is the belly which is attacked, and the poison eats it way right through the flesh into the entrails ... the cartilage of the labourers noses was being eaten away by foul gases ... all for fourpence an hour.

This was the time when the pioneering Elsie Inglis received her doctorate of medicine in Edinburgh and shortly afterwards was appointed lecturer in gynaecology at Edinburgh Medical College for Women, which she had helped found with her father. She now began her battle against the grinding poverty and chronic sickness endemic in the Edinburgh tenement buildings.

Within the nursing system, Ethel Fenwick and her cohorts continued their fight for change and improvements. During the 1899 London meeting of the Congress of the International Council of Women, Ethel had been appointed Treasurer of the Congress funds. One whole day of the Congress was devoted to the nursing issues, and her friend Mrs Sewall was the conference chairman. Distinguished nurses from America, Denmark, Holland, and Cape Colony attended Congress and the nursing section was the very first international gathering of nurses. Naturally, state registration and women's suffrage was discussed. Florence Nightingale, then aged 80, sent the assembled nurses a letter of support:

> *Dear Nurses – very dear nurses,*
>
> *Thank you, thank you for all the progress you have made these last years. May God bless you, and He does bless you, you should be the salt of the earth, for such opportunities are yours for showing in your practice what women should be. And that every year should show this more and more, is the earnest prayer of your affectionate and grateful,*
> *Florence Nightingale*

Ethel Fenwick proposed steps be taken to found an International Council of Nurses. Since nurses from other countries were still in London, they were invited to attend the annual meeting of the Matrons' Council. This was held the day following the Congress, at the Matron's House in St Bartholomew's. (This house was destroyed by a flying bomb in the Second World War.) And so, on 1 July 1899, at the meeting of the Matrons' Council of Great Britain and Ireland, Mrs Fenwick made her inspiring address on international cooperation. Stressing the need for professional education and organisation, the need to unite with delegates from Nursing Councils of all nations, she ended by proposing:

> That steps be taken to organize an International Council of Nurses ... It has for some time been felt that an International Congress of Nurses is greatly wanted, in order to elicit the views of women engaged in the work, in every part of the world, upon the fundamental principles of the organization of their profession.

So it was that the long-held dream of an International Council of Nurses was founded – to promote international cooperation between nurses and to provide opportunities to meet and discuss professional issues. Structure of the International Council of Nurses was based on that of the ICW membership by being restricted to one national association from each country. The individual national associations would consist of representatives of various self-governing nurses organisations of each country.

Voting papers had been sent to all the Provisional Committee members. Ethel Fenwick was elected President, holding that post for the first five years. Lavinia Dock of the USA was elected Secretary, a post she held for twenty-two years. Miss Snively of Canada was elected Treasurer. At this meeting, it was agreed to accept the invitation of the Buffalo Nurses' Association to hold a Congress there in 1901. A year later, on 5 July 1900, the British members of the Provisional

Committee met to discuss the draft constitution they had created for this International Council of Nurses.

For the first twelve years, the offices of the International Council of Nurses were at the office of the Registered Nurses' Society in Oxford Street, London. (The RNS was a non-profit making society, set up by Mrs Fenwick for private nurses who were members of the RBNA.) This was the very first international organisation of a group of professional women in the world. It was the culminating event of a momentous century which had seen the transformation of nursing from an occupation for the destitute and degraded to a profession for the educated. Although the powerful primary impulse was due to the charisma of Florence Nightingale, its development into its modern form, through national and international organisation, can only be attributed to the hard work of the indomitable Ethel Fenwick.

Chapter 6

# The New Era: Some Success 1900–1909

At the beginning of the twentieth century, only 5 per cent of the British population were aged 65 or older; by the beginning of the twenty-first century, this figure had risen to 17 per cent. The average twentieth-century household consisted of 4.5 people; by the start of the twenty-first century, it was a mere 2.3 individuals. In the beginning of the twentieth century, only 5 per cent were single households; a century later this had risen to 33 per cent. Agricultural workers once accounted for 12 per cent of the working population, but within 100 years this had fallen to 2 per cent; office workers, once 18 per cent, rose to become 40 per cent of the workforce. Despite more leisure time, church attendance had fallen.

Equality for women was a distant objective; even by the end of the twentieth century the United Nations calculated that, of all the work hours in the world, women did 80 per cent but received only 10 per cent of world income and controlled less than 1 per cent of world resources.

Many changes occurred during Ethel Fenwick's lifetime in spite of, or perhaps because of, the several serious outbreaks of war and the consequent requirements for adaptation and survival. The impetus for change continued to gather momentum in every direction as the twentieth century began, although medicine and public health issues still had a long way to go. The start of 1900 was heralded by a massive outbreak of influenza during the peak of which, in London alone, fifty people were dying daily. The school in the Moray village of Fochabers, Milne's Institute, was closed for two weeks in October due to an outbreak of diphtheria.

The Boer War (1899–1902) was going badly and in Moray, Ethel's county of birth, the local paper, *The Northern Scot*, reported hundreds of locals turning out to see off the regiment of Seaforth soldiers as they were setting out to the South African war:

> The enthusiasm shown in Elgin on Wednesday last on the occasion of the departure of the Volunteers chosen to represent the 3rd battalion of the Seaforths was unprecedented. Early in the day people began to gather in clusters in front of the Orderly Room and the Drill Hall, and as the day advanced the crowd increased, being largely augmented by country people, until by 3 pm many hundreds were waiting on the High Street. The men were drawn up in a line four deep, the two front lines being composed of those who were destined for the front forthwith, while the two back lines made up the reserves. During the interval of preparation for the farewell ceremonial, the pipe band discoursed stirring music which was greatly enjoyed. When the train steamed slowly out of the Highland Railway Station, bearing away the brave lads who are to fight for their Queen and country in South Africa, the scene, even in the semi-darkness, was singularly striking and memorable.

In the same edition of the paper was the following interesting, alarmist medical advertisement:

> While everyone's attention is directed to the War in South Africa, we are apt to forget that a war is constantly raging within our own bodies. The germs of disease are ever striving to obtain mastery over the healthy organisms, so that if we have, say a cough or cold and we leave it to cure itself, the chances are that it will run on and on, from bad to worse, ending very probably in consumption. This is why I draw your attention to Smiths Brothers' famous compound essence of linseed. It is a marvelous remedy, and has cured hundreds throughout Elgin and Morayshire. To be had only from R. Halley, chemist, Gordon Arms Buildings, Elgin.

Britain rejoiced at the news of the relief of Ladysmith, in March 1900, after four months of siege. The British forces led by Lord Dundonald, with Winston Churchill by his side, entered Ladysmith on the afternoon of 1 March 1900. There was more rejoicing later at news of the relief of Mafeking in May by Major General Robert Baden Powell, following a siege which had begun the previous October. *The Northern Scot* reported the local June celebrations of the relief of Mafeking, which included a firework display in nearby Lossiemouth square, hometown to Ramsay MacDonald:

> During the rejoicing in Lossiemouth in connection with the relief of Mafeking, a fireworks display was held in the Square where a large crowd had gathered – but rogue fireworks went off in the wrong direction and injured a number of people. Such was the extent of the injuries that some casualties had to have limbs amputated, and one lad later died in hospital.

The British nation was shocked by the horrific news of the Boxer rebellion in China in May 1900. The rebellion was anti-foreign and anti-Christian, and resulted in hundreds of missionaries and their families being slain. Foreigners were killed and converts to Christianity were beheaded by fanatics. 'Boxers' was a name that foreigners gave to a Chinese secret society which practised certain boxing and calisthenic rituals in the belief that this gave them supernatural powers, making them impervious to bullets. The objective of the rebels was the destruction of the current dynasty and elimination of the corrupt and corrupting influence of westerners.

In response to the crisis, a hastily organised group of troops comprising American, British, Russian, French, and Italian soldiers was sent to China. The American men were dispatched in winter uniforms, and the Russians forgot their cannon. By August 1900, when these allies had entered Peking, westerners sheltering in the embassies and foreign legations there had endured a fifty-six-day siege and were down to their last week of supplies.

Within British society, attitudes remained hypocritical and inflexible towards some aspects of self-expression and in 1900 the great writer Oscar Wilde died in Paris at the early age of 46 in disgrace and abject poverty. He had served a two-year prison sentence of hard labour when convicted for homosexuality, after which he was a broken man. In spite of his wit, talent, and initial popularity, Wilde had always been perceived as a middle-class Irishman. His lover, the spoilt and vicious second son of the Marquis of Queensbury, escaped prosecution when the Victorian upper classes closed ranks to protect one of their own.

Charities continued to flourish, education and self-improvement were encouraged and Scots-born industrialist and philanthropist, Andrew Carnegie, established public library buildings in England, Scotland, and the United States between 1900 and 1917. In all of them an 'open access' policy was adopted, making information as well as literary entertainment available to everyone.

In reaction to so many representations of classical art, Art Nouveau began to flourish and quickly became popularised when it appeared on magazine covers. Early cinema began when Thomas Edison invented a kinetoscope that projected film onto walls, providing much more convenient viewing than bending over to look into a wooden case as had been previously necessary. Having mastered the art of riding the bicycle, women were beginning to enjoy escalation of more social freedom and independence – a development that would prove to be vital for future workers such as district nurses and midwives.

The year 1900, which saw the birth of Elizabeth Bowes-Lyon, was the one in which development of the telephone was accelerated and long-distance calls became possible. This was also the year that saw the wave of labour strikes begun by coal miners on the Continent spread to other workers, including steelworkers and glassblowers. All were all demanding pay increases, an eight-hour day, and better working conditions. British Trade Unions created the Labour party. In July, the progressive British Parliament passed a new labour act which included outlawing child labour, allowing workers' compensation, and covering for illness.

Eating habits changed following the development, by the Kellogg brothers, of a method of producing crunchy flakes of processed grain and the subsequent creation of the Kellogg's Toasted Corn Flakes company. The Marmite Food Extract company was formed in 1902, converting yeast protein into a palatable food. With the discovery of vitamins, Marmite was found to be the richest source of the vitamin B complex and as such was to prove a valuable as well as popular addition to the British diet.

A tale of mixed opportunism and inspired entrepreneurship is worth a brief mention here, if only to further illustrate the spirit of the age. James 'Scotty' Phillip, born in Dallas near Elgin, Moray, had emigrated to America and enjoyed a variety of work including scout, cowboy, and miner. He married a native American wife, the half-sister of the famous Crazy Horse, who was one of the last great warrior-chiefs, instrumental in defeating General Custer at the battle of Little Bighorn. As well as becoming one of the first senators of Dakota and running a vast cattle ranch, Scotty Phillip established a post office in a South Dakota town which now bears his name.

Following the slaughter of over 60 million buffalo for sport during the days of the 'wild west', Scotty Phillip kept part of the Indian heritage alive by creating a sanctuary in 1899. By his actions, he managed to save the last of the American buffalo, providing the bloodline for every beast in today's sanctuaries. When he died suddenly of cerebral haemorrhage in 1911, people travelled for three days to attend his funeral – a special train had to be laid on for his mourners and it was recorded that the buffalo came down from the hill pasture to watch his funeral taking place in the cemetery beside the sanctuary.

Progress in nursing reform continued. As well as the need for a professional education and organisation, Ethel Fenwick believed that, since the aims of nurses all over the world were the same, they should unite to form a body, with delegations from the Nursing Councils of all nations. She believed that 'Professions, like nations, only flourish by the development of an individual sense of responsibility. The first aim, therefore, of the International Council of Nurses, is to organise Nurses all the world over, and to make them articulate.'

The original Constitution survived, with only minor alterations, until 1965. Membership of the ICN is limited to one nursing organisation per nation. Nowadays every member country provides a nurse – usually the President – to serve on the Council of National Representatives and this Council determines the policies of the ICN, which meets every two years. The Council of National Representatives elects a Board of Directors, which in turn elects the Administrative and Finance Committee, which handles the budget for the ICN. In addition, two standing Committees report to the Council of National Representatives; one reporting on education, nursing practice, social and economic welfare of nurses, the other investigating the eligibility of organisations for joining the International Council and also reviews the status of members, giving help and advice to countries wishing to join. The headquarters of the ICN is now in Geneva, facilitating its work in conjunction with the World Health Organization.

Medicine at the turn of the century had made major advances – but much more lay ahead. Like most of the population, doctors were relatively poor. In contrast to the large practices of today, they worked on their own and were consulted only when patients were very ill. Life expectancy was around fifty, and about one in eight children died before their first birthday. The average weekly wage for a farm worker was 17/6. Many people belonged to a provident club that paid a local doctor an annual fee of around 4/-. A house call cost 2/6d and a visit to the doctor's surgery would cost about 1/6d. The doctor would dispense medicine himself, which would be inclusive in the fee; the fouler the taste, the more efficacious the medicine was believed to be.

An incredible array of concoctions were used for medicine. Arsenic was considered a near panacea for all ills, and croton oil (a violent laxative) was used to treat mental disorders. Malaria was cured with quinine and was the only infectious disease that was treatable. Smallpox was the only vaccination available; insulin was unknown and tobacco smoking was recommended for asthmatics. Pain was treated with either aspirin or morphine, with nothing available in between for controlling moderate pain. The technique of appendicectomy was new and the operation was often performed on a kitchen table. In retrospect, a well-scrubbed kitchen table would have been safer than the available operating theatres in those days! Nothing more sophisticated than the rag and bottle application of anaesthesia was used. Antenatal care was unknown, and death in childbirth was a common hazard, women being 200 times more likely to die in childbirth than nowadays. Many babies did not survive to their second birthday. Doctors were never sued, despite inadvertently killing many of their patients.

In the days before the National Health Service, when many were afraid of the expense of calling out a doctor, folk would try many strange remedies. Within living memory, a farm servant had to have a leg amputation following attempts to cure a wound infection by applying cow dung. Bone-setters, precursors of the modern chiropractor, were much sought after – often best visited in the morning when they were gentler in their operations. It was well known that, following a liquid lunch, the more intemperate practitioners perceived less pain themselves, and were consequently far more vigorous in their treatment!

Britain was plunged into mourning in 1901 when, at the age of 82, Queen Victoria died.

Movements for change, begun in the final decades of the nineteenth century, were gaining momentum. Ethel Fenwick wrote in an editorial in the *Nursing Record*, 21 September 1901:

> The era of the 'ministering angel' and the silly sentimentality inseparable from that aspect of the work, which did so much harm, has, we hope, as completely passed as the days and degradation for-ever associated with Sairey Gamp. The era of the trained nurse

as a woman desirous to do the best professional work in her power has dawned...

Following her trip to America and her visits to hospitals there, Ethel Fenwick was busily involved with the new International Council of Nurses. In arranging for the ICN Congress in Buffalo in 1901, she advised nurses intending to travel there, 'If you wish to have peace on board do not mention that you are a nurse.' Sound advice and still relevant, as any nurse can attest today! By 1905, the cost of a transatlantic third-class liner ticket to America had increased to £6.

The Pan-American exposition was held in 1901 in Buffalo, New York and the International Council of Nurses first held their meeting there in September to coincide with this massive event. Ethel Fenwick organised a part of the exposition, delivered a presidential address and addressed a meeting of nearly 2,000 nurses on the need for higher education of nurses.

The Congress in Buffalo was overshadowed by President McKinley's assassination, but 500–600 nurses attended daily. As membership of the ICN was by national organisation only, Ethel Fenwick founded the National Council of Nurses in order to enable England to be represented at the 1904 Conference to be held in Berlin. Following a speech from Ethel Fenwick, a resolution was passed in favour of registration. At that time, in 1901, South Africa was the only country which had nurse registration.

It wasn't all hard work for Ethel – she and her husband would travel by train to Cumbria to spend summer holidays at Dunningwell with her sister and brother-in-law Clara and Charlie Myers. After her marriage, Clara had persuaded her husband Charles to build a new home on the estate. In the 1890s, this had been considered a very modern establishment as it had bathrooms for the servants as well as a bathroom in Charles's dressing room – but at that time it had no electricity. The 1901 census records 57-year-old Charles Myers, retired army officer, as head of the household, living at Dunningwell with 46-year-old Clara, his wife, and 70-year-old Harriet Storer, his mother-in-law, 'Living on own Means'. The 44-year-old cook and two housemaids in their twenties were also recorded as living there.

Ethel, her husband and son were just some of the many assorted family members who descended upon Dunningwell for the annual gathering in the summer holidays. The four acres of garden and fifteen acres of woodland provided plenty of room for visitors to wander and there were plenty of country walks surrounding the nearby village. Ethel enjoyed brisk, refreshing country walks around the estate and country lanes, accompanied by family and their various dogs.

Theodore Roosevelt was sworn in as 26th President of the United States following the assassination of President McKinley. That same year, the Gillette Safety Razor Company was founded, and America watched in amazement as Carrie Nation, armed with a hatchet, led an unrelenting crusade against alcohol in Kansas. The movement for prohibition of alcohol was gaining a fierce and frenzied momentum.

The leaders of the Chinese Boxer rebellion were executed. Becqueral discovered the internal structure of atoms and Marconi managed to send the first Atlantic message from Poldhu in Cornwall to St John's, Newfoundland. Having been influenced and inspired in his humanitarian work by Florence Nightingale, Jean Dunant, founder of the Red Cross, shared the first Nobel peace prize with Frederick Passy. The first Nobel prize for physics was awarded to Wilhelm Roentgen following his discovery of X-rays.

Medical research continued to progress and another important medical breakthrough was made when yellow fever was found to be carried by mosquitoes. One of the researchers, 25-year-old American army nurse Clara Maas, died in August 1901 after voluntarily contracting the disease. Once American army pathologist and bacteriologist Walter Reed had proved the source of the infection, official action by military engineers in 1901 to eradicate mosquitoes freed Havana from the disease within ninety days. This enabled work on building the Panama Canal to begin successfully in 1902.

In December 1901, David Lloyd George made a dramatic escape from an enraged Birmingham mob who were protesting at his stance against the Boer War. Lloyd George had made previous attacks on Colonial Secretary Joseph Chamberlain, accusing him of personally profiting from the war through his connection with armaments firms. The mob threw bottles and bricks and smashed windows, and Lloyd George was only able to escape by disguising himself in a policeman's coat and helmet. However, the tide of public opinion was turning. The Boer guerrillas began to be admired for their courage while emerging reports of Kitchener's policy of incarcerating Boer wives and families in concentration camps shocked public opinion into a change of attitude. Reports by Emily Hobhouse about the lack of hygiene and medical facilities in these camps, revealing devastating mortality levels of around 28,000 prisoners, caused outrage. Lloyd George's opinions were no longer seen as unpatriotic and he became a celebrity.

The following year, 1902, saw the introduction of the Midwives Act. Midwives finally achieved education, examination, licence, and registration. Undoubtedly a major factor in their achievement of regulation and registration was that their work took place in the community, affected most families and their mistakes and inefficiencies were obvious to all. The need for regulation was incontrovertible. The new Midwives Act allowed the setting up of a Central Midwives Board. From then on, no woman could habitually, or for gain, practice midwifery except under the direction of a doctor, unless she was certified by the Board. Nurses faced a much harder struggle for registration.

In June 1902, with Ethel Fenwick as secretary and treasurer, the Matrons' Council of Britain launched the Society for the State Registration of Nurses. Within a year, they had 900 members and put forward the first Bill for registration of nurses. The tide was running in their favour. However, there were several serious opponents – Matron of the London hospital, Eva Luckes, being the main one. She was now an implacable enemy of the cause that the Fenwicks held so dear. Eva Luckes firmly believed State Registration would degrade the high art of nursing to the status of a mere profession and thought that for some nurses 'a little training goes a long way', adding 'a pseudoscientific person is most objectionable in the sickroom'. Miss Luckes was much admired and supported by Florence Nightingale for her vocational attitude but between her and Ethel Fenwick there was a vast disparity of opinion which allowed for no compromise.

Although the British Medical Association supported registration, the Clerk of the Society of Apothecaries, fearing that nurses might set up in opposition to doctors, added his thoughts on the matter of nurse registration: 'Speaking for myself, I never saw such a thing as a nurse inside my house. Now my boy has hardly anything the matter with him before in comes a nurse ... I think there is a good deal of unnecessary fuss made in these days about illness.'

The first Bill for registration of nurses, drafted by Mrs and Dr Bedford Fenwick and Isla Stewart, had been put forward in 1902 and was introduced as Private Member's Bill in February 1904. At the same time, a second Bill on behalf of the Royal British Nurses' Association for the registration of nurses was promoted in the Commons. The Royal British Nurses' Association was still under the control of the Fenwicks' opponents, and although they were now supporting registration, Ethel did not trust them and labelled their bill the 'employers' bill'. Both Bills sought to establish a central nursing council to be responsible for the system of registration, but they differed in the proposed composition of the council. The Fenwicks gave a majority of the seats on the council to nurses, but the Royal British Nurses' Association Bill gave hospital and medical authorities the controlling vote. Both parties lobbied MPs to gain support, and eventually, after months of campaigning, the House of Commons appointed a Select Committee to consider the expediency of providing for a register of nurses.

The first pure hormone to be isolated from natural sources, adrenaline, was isolated from the suprarenal gland by a Japanese biochemist, Jokichi Takamine. Having graduated from the Imperial University of Tokyo, Takamine had done post-graduate studies at Glasgow and later visited the United States. He eventually settled in America, where his pioneering research in the isolation of adrenaline was carried out. He continued his close ties with Japan, being involved with industrial developments including that of the manufacture of Bakelite.

The end of the Boer War was a great relief to the British public, who were finally becoming aware of the horrors involved. The Boer and the Boxer wars had cost one-third of the United Kingdom's annual budget and 100,000 British lives had been lost in the Boer War alone. While the Boer menfolk were fighting a guerrilla war, over 26,000 of their women and children had died in the concentration camps set up by the British for Boer civilians. The death rate in the camps continued to rise as a result of a measles epidemic compounded by neglect and inadequate feeding. Peace was finally negotiated in 1902.

After a sports car had reached the incredible speed of 62mph, one of the big questions of the day was about fuel: which would dominate the future – steam or gasoline? In Europe, fashionable women were wearing hats so heavy they needed to be wedged on with false hair and held with hat pins – while the hardy and practical women of Australia attained the vote. In America, the suffragette leader Elizabeth Cady Stanton died aged 86 and in Britain Emmeline Pankhurst founded the Women's Social and Political Union to promote enfranchisement of women.

Edward VII was crowned on 9 August 1902, the ceremony having been delayed for six weeks due to his appendicectomy. Luckily the new developments in anaesthetic and antisepsis techniques meant such operations no longer resulted in a high mortality rate. In a radical operation under the supervision of Lord Lister, Edward's infected abscess was drained successfully and the next day he was sitting up in bed and smoking a cigar. Two weeks later, he was pronounced to be out of danger and as a reward his surgeon, Sir Edward Treeves, was created a Baronet.

The health of the general population remained poor – it was recorded that two out of every five men volunteering for the army were unfit for recruitment. Dentistry became more popular when porcelain was used for the first time for filling teeth. The new Gillette Safety Razor Company sold 168 razors in 1902 – but a year later sold 15 million of the revolutionary devices, and the Ford company sold its first automobile, the 'model A', in Detroit. A message via the New Pacific Cable could now circle the globe in just under ten minutes, heralding the age of almost instant communication. Marie Curie became the first woman permitted to attend a meeting of the Royal Institute in London in 1903 when her husband was a lecturer there. In Edinburgh, in 1904, appalled at the ignorant prejudices against women within her own profession, Dr Elsie Inglis founded a maternity hospice for the poor, completely staffed by women, and the forerunner of a later women's hospital. The issue of women's health in childbirth was beginning to be addressed seriously at last, although it was to take a long time for women's opinions on the subject to be treated with respect by the authoritarian medical establishment.

Reforms were under way and the Liberal government was fighting poverty by bringing in many social improvements including the introduction of free school meals, old age pensions, and labour exchanges. Winston Churchill left the Tory party, joined the Liberals in 1904 and was elected MP for Manchester.

Meantime, at an International Council of Nurses meeting in Berlin 1904, Ethel Fenwick retired as president and was elected honorary vice-president with a seat on the grand council. The first three national councils, those of Great Britain and Ireland, the USA, and Germany had been set up by this date. Ethel Fenwick had been elected president of the National Council of Trained Nurses of Great Britain and Ireland, which represented fifteen affiliated nursing organisations.

At the Berlin Congress, the ICN adopted Ethel's *British Journal of Nursing* as its official journal. This had originally been the *Nursing Record*, which Ethel Fenwick had renamed in 1902, and through which she aimed to reach all English-speaking nurses all over the world. She was influenced by the *American Journal of Nursing*, with which her friend Lavina Dock was associated, and the aims of the two journals were identical.

While the great Russian physiologist Ivan Pavlov was awarded the Nobel Prize for Physiology for his work on digestive secretion, Russia and Japan were at war over dominance of Korea and Manchuria. Following growing unrest within his country, Czar Nicolas proposed reforms but these were too little and too late. Mistaking it for a Japanese warship, in the heat of the moment the Russian Baltic fleet sunk a British fishing boat in the North Sea in the area of Dogger Bank in October 1904. British warships were sent to surround the Russians and relations between the two countries were very tense until an international commission was appointed to examine the circumstances of the attack.

In urban America, the New York Subway was opened in 1904 but, in the state of Georgia, desperate farmers resorted to burning two million bales of cotton in order to prop up falling prices. In the same state, two black men were dragged from court and burnt at the stake. In spite of the racial intolerance in his country, George Washington Carver, born to slaves in Missouri in 1861, became a chemist and botanist. Obtaining an MA in agriculture, he eventually developed new uses for soya beans, sweet potatoes, peanuts, and other crops and was a prime catalyst in revitalising agriculture in the southern states.

An outbreak of at least fifty-one cases of typhoid, which resulted in at least three deaths, was traced to a carrier, Mary Mallon, who was a cook working around the Oyster Bay and Long Island area in America. Although a carrier, she was immune to the typhoid bacillus. After the outbreak had been traced to her, Mary, nicknamed Typhoid Mary, disappeared and the long hunt for her by the public health authorities began.

Problems in Russia persisted with the incidents in 1905 of 'Bloody Sunday' in St Petersburg when troops opened fire and killed 500 people, and the mutiny of the crew on the battleship *Potemkin* during which the captain was killed. After much negotiation, American intervention and mediation by President Theodore Roosevelt, the Russo-Japanese peace talks ended in a treaty and the Russians withdrew from Manchuria.

There was good news for the reformers in nursing. In 1905, having discussed and supported the issue for some years, a Committee of the British Medical Association recommend registration of nurses. This Select Committee had taken evidence from thirty-three witnesses including the Bedford Fenwicks, Sir Henry Burdett, Sydney Holland, Eva Luckes, and Isla Stewart. When giving evidence before the Committee, Eva Luckes was asked if she thought that working 14 hours day every day of the week was too much for the ordinary woman. This intractable Matron replied, 'I do not think a nurse is an ordinary woman, or she would not have chosen work which taxes her feelings and energies, mental and physical, so much.'

It would appear that adverse comments made in the *Nursing Record* about the exploitation of London nurses were not so libellous after all!

Sir Victor Horsley responded to concerns that the registration of nurses would not ensure a nurse remained competent:

> That contention is absurd, because the same applied to the registration of every professional man. If an individual has gone through a long course of professional training to acquire expert knowledge, that individual is justified in requiring from the State the registration of the fact, and unless the individual misbehaves in any way, that registration remains good.

Once registration had been approved by the Committee, Ethel Fenwick and her supporters were now convinced that statutory recognition of their profession could no longer be postponed – but sadly they had overestimated the influence of a Select Committee report. Opposition remained strong. Two Registration Bills were reintroduced to the House of Commons in 1906 and 1907 by private members, without government support, and each time they were blocked by opponents of registration.

Professional recognition for the nurses was not the only area of reform to suffer setbacks. From 1906 onwards, seven suffrage bills were defeated in Parliament. Understandably, many suffragists became more inclined to acts of violence in order to draw attention to their cause.

Nurses were not the only people demanding changes. The new Edwardian age was politically turbulent. In England and Wales, the numbers of people receiving poor relief had increased to 800,000, while 250,000 were reduced to living in the dreaded workhouses. One of the most important social changes was that of attitude. Public perceptions had altered and a more compassionate and understanding mood prevailed as poverty was perceived to be a misfortune instead of being due to laziness. Reforms were under way and the Liberal government was fighting poverty by bringing in many social improvements including the introduction of free school meals, old age pensions, and labour exchanges.

While the Suffragette movement escalated in London, Amundson succeeded in finding the magnetic Pole and Einstein proposed his theory of relativity. Medical knowledge continued to expand. After tests carried out by J. Goldberger on Mississippi goal inmates, Pellagra, (now known to be a result of lack of vitamin B), was found to be caused by poor diet. Dr Robert Koch received the Nobel prize for medicine for his earlier discovery of the bacillus that causes tuberculosis. His work had been made possible thanks to the discovery of aniline dyes to stain bacteria, and the use of agar (discovered by his laboratory assistant Angelina Hesse) as a medium to grow bacteria. From then on it was possible to use the same technique to discover initially the cholera bacteria and eventually many more.

Progress occurred on the domestic front with the development in 1906 of a washing machine which promised to do in three or four hours the same amount of washing that would take two full days by hand. Vacuum cleaners were still in their infancy, requiring two people to operate. However, demonstrations of their capabilities in places such as Buckingham Palace, Westminster Abbey, and Windsor Palace were impressive, even although police were called after a demonstration of the new machine had been held at the Royal Mint. Apparently, the demonstrators had inadvertently sucked up a quantity of gold dust!

In Ethel's home district of Moray, electricity was introduced to the village of Fochabers in 1906, thanks to the generosity of the 7th Duke of Richmond and Gordon. Fochabers had electric lighting before its larger neighbour, Elgin. The switching on was ceremoniously marked by a pipe-band and a dance, as water from the river Spey was used to drive a turbine which generated electricity. In cold weather, a man was employed to go around the streets at night ringing a bell to warn when there was ice on the water, which blocked the turbine, with his cry of 'Nae licht the nicht' (No light tonight).

In 1906, J. F. Smith, president of the Mormon Church, was charged with polygamy after the birth of his 43rd child – born to his fifth wife. Several American states had already given women the vote, but suffragettes were still active in France. Although Madame Curie became the first woman to teach at the Sorbonne, her nomination for the French Academy was defeated by one vote because she was female. Drawing support from all classes, Dr Elsie Inglis founded the Scottish Women's Suffrage Federation, and became its secretary. Emmeline Pankhurst caused much controversy when she forecast that violence might be needed in the struggle for female emancipation.

After being constructed in a mere fourteen months, the largest battleship, and the world's fastest warship, the *Dreadnaught*, was launched in Portsmouth, achieving a speed of 21 knots during speed trails and marking the start of a naval arms race between Britain and Germany. Winston Churchill led protests about the excessive noise produced by the modern traffic.

A report from the Boer War Commission revealed that incompetence and corruption throughout the conduct of the war had cost over one million pounds. Hundreds of people died as a consequence of the natural disasters which occurred with the eruption of Vesuvius and with the San

Francisco earthquake. The Russian peasants' revolt was a forerunner of a much larger man-made disaster.

An international health organisation was established in Paris in 1907 with the aim of acquiring and transmitting information of serious communicable diseases from participating nations, and to study and develop sanitary conventions and quarantine regulations on shipping and train travel.

Doctors pontificated on many subjects; at a BMA conference, it was declared that children must be stopped from smoking as it was undoubtedly harmful and the Children's Act 1908 made it an offence for persons under 16 years of age to be sold or to buy cigarettes or cigarette papers. Sadly, less notice was taken of this advice than of the theories of a certain Professor W. I. Thomas. In 1907, this medical sage wrote a book, *Sex & Society*, in which he placed women on an intellectual par with savages. He did, however, acknowledge that the American woman had made an approach towards the standards of professional scholarship and that 'a number of women of natural ability and character are realising some definite aim'. He nevertheless considered these as sporadic cases.

That same year, women in Finland won their first seats in Parliament after Finland had been the first European country to give women the vote in 1906. In Norway, a woman was entitled to vote as long as she, or her husband, was a regular tax payer. In Britain, suffragettes and their supporters stormed Parliament. Sixty were arrested and many were hurt as a consequence of alleged police brutality.

A new form of protest germinated in South Africa when a young lawyer, by the name of Gandhi, urged civil disobedience in protest against the Asiatic Registration Bill. More serious trouble occurred in Vancouver, British Columbia, when 10,000 labourers protested against the government's encouragement of immigrants. The ensuing riots drove 2,000 Chinese from their homes and other anti-Oriental riots took place in America. Meanwhile, an uprising in China saw nationalists demanding land redistribution and a republic. Suffragettes began their United States campaign with a big rally in New York, which was supported by many men. In Britain in 1907, Keir Hardie's Women's Enfranchisement Bill was defeated.

In America, health authorities led by George Soper, a sanitary engineer in the New York City Department of Health, finally caught up with Typhoid Mary, who was again working as a cook. Once more she escaped, but was eventually caught and, for public safety, was committed to an isolation centre on North Brother Island, off the Bronx. There, despite an appeal to the US Supreme Court, she stayed – but only for four years.

During this time, the stalwart founders of the International Council of Nurses were cementing relationships between nurses from all over the world, using social occasions and publicity to keep the spirit and enthusiasm of members alight. In 1907, Isla Stewart and Ethel Fenwick went to Paris to make arrangements for an International Congress of Nurses which was to hold an interim conference there later that year. There they met Mlle Chaptal, who was later to become president of the National Association of Trained Nurses of France and also of the ICN. Through her influence, the British nurses secured the interest of the Director General of the Assistance Publique, who gave them every assistance and agreed to open the Nurses' Congress. Ever mindful of the importance of good publicity, Ethel gave an International Press dinner. She summarised her views in a speech at the Council:

> To enumerate our most pressing needs, we require preliminary education before entering hospital wards; we need post-graduate education to keep us in the running; we need special instruction as teachers to fit us for the responsible positions of sisters and superintendents; we need a State-constituted board to examine and maintain discipline in our ranks, and we must have legal status to protect our professional rights and to ensure us ample professional autonomy.

In America in 1908, thousands of women marched through New York demanding shorter hours, and better pay. The marchers were condemning child labour, poor and unsafe working conditions, and demanding that women were given the right to vote. In Georgia prohibition (of alcohol) was introduced, while in New York a Miss Katie Mulchey was arrested for smoking in public and, being unable to pay the fine, she was jailed. The Olympic games were held in pouring rain in London, with the Irish contingent incensed at competing under the British flag, and the Finns refusing to carry the Russian flag.

Now at a price affordable to the masses, the first Model T rolled off the Ford production line in Detroit to be known with affection as the Tin Lizzy. Toothpaste appeared in a tube when Colgate produced Colgate Ribbon Dental Cream. Acutely aware of the disadvantages of being vertically challenged, the Japanese made an effort to grow into a taller nation by encouraging less sitting about and more exercise, while doctors in New York saved a man's life by sewing up a stab wound in his heart. Following the success of several new surgical techniques, the Head of the Rockefeller Institute for Medical Research made the apparently ludicrous prediction that transplants to replace diseased organs in humans would be possible in the future. The surgeon who was to pioneer the technique of heart and lung transplants was not born until fourteen years after this dogmatic pronouncement.

In January 1908, Ethel's mother, 78-year-old Harriette, died at Clara's home at Dunningwell and was taken to be buried alongside her husband, in the churchyard of St Helena's at Thoroton, Nottinghamshire.

The third Bill for registration was promoted in February 1908, this time in the House of Lords by the Central Hospital Council for London, representing the London General hospitals. It proposed the establishment of an official directory of nurses, to be maintained by an official register. However, there was no provision for self-government of nurses and no minimum standard of training laid down. Ethel Fenwick was incensed and called it the 'Nurses' Enslavement Bill' and urged all nurses to protest against this piece of reactionary legislation.

The Bill was lost on its second reading in the House of Lords and this was interpreted as a sign of support by the registration lobby.

Consequently, they withdrew their Bill from the Commons and introduced it instead in the Lords. The Bill was passed in the Lords, but without government support it failed to get a reading in the Commons. These complicated legislative convolutions must have been incredibly frustrating for supporters of reform.

Ethel Fenwick was not just concerned with registration for nurses. She was an ardent supporter of women's suffrage and, recognising there could be no responsibility or power without the vote, did her utmost to make nurses aware of the issues involved. She was the nursing representative on the Committee of the National Union of Women's Suffrage Societies, and led the nurses marching in the great 'Suffrage Sunday' procession of June 1908.

The 'Suffrage Sunday' procession was a momentous event, drawing 15,000 women from all over the country. The *British Journal of Nursing* issued marching orders and directives urging those women incapable of walking to follow in a brake at 10d a seat and telling them where to obtain ribbon or scarves in the suffrage colours of white, green and purple. It was a great occasion; the procession had seventy banners carried by women graduates, doctors, writers, artists, pharmacists, typists, shop assistants, and factory workers. The nurses were all in outdoor uniform, and marched behind a banner of rose satin emblazoned in gold with the name of Florence Nightingale and a lighthouse. This highly successful gathering raised high hopes for votes for women, but there were to be years of painful struggle ahead, and a wait nearly as long as that of the nurses for State Registration.

The British establishment was shaken in October 1908 when 10,000 protesters stormed Parliament demanding votes for women and one bold woman actually managed to reach the door of the House of Commons. She was carried out by three men and immediately afterwards an order was passed forbidding women access to the building. Twenty-four suffragettes and twelve people protesting about unemployment were jailed as a consequence of this alarming threat to democracy.

Perceptive politicians could sense forthcoming problems elsewhere. King Edward went to Germany to meet up with Kaiser Wilhelm and in 1908 Sir Edward Grey, the British Foreign Secretary wrote to a friend:

> The German Emperor … he is like a battleship with steam up and screws going, but with no rudder and he will run into something one day and cause a catastrophe. He has made a fool of Germany and all the world is laughing at him and the Germans do not like being laughed at … Germany is very strong and very restless, like a person whose boots are too small for him. I don't think there will be a war at present, but it will be difficult to keep the peace for another five years.

In January 1909 the first payments of a British Old Age pension were made. Anyone over 70 years of age whose income was under £21 a year received 5/- a week. The growing recreational activity for rich Europeans was going on the African safari, preferably to shoot and kill as many large animals as possible. The Balkans were in turmoil, and there was unease and trepidation throughout Europe when Germany revealed an ability to build big battleships very rapidly.

Apache warrior and leader, Geronimo, died aged 80 having fought many battles and witnessed massacres and betrayal of his people. In his later years, he was given permission by the War Department to earn money by selling photographs and handicrafts at expositions – a sad and undignified ending for a great leader of his time. Bleriot flew across the Channel and Robert Peary, along with his black assistant, Matthew Henson, reached the North Pole after a 36-day trek. In Italy an international rescue operation was mounted after the horrendous Messina earthquake resulted in 200,000 deaths.

Emmeline Pankhurst travelled to New York to speak at a rally in the Carnegie Hall and American Carrie Chapman presided at a convention in London of the International Women's Alliance. It was a time when many American wives were being deserted and left to bring up families alone. Alcohol was recognised as a major factor in the desertion statistics and it was obvious that desertion was cheaper than divorce. Young women went to work in factories in order to support their families and this was blamed for the erosion of domestic skills. As well as women's suffrage, child labour was becoming an issue of concern in America. A National Negro Committee was founded to press for suffrage and an end to racial prejudice. The trustees of Harvard University decided to exclude an application by Inez Mulholland as they 'feared a drop in applicants because of prejudice against females and males studying together'. One trustee admitted his opposition to all change – including railroads and the telegraph.

In April 1909, Ethel rallied her supporters to take their places in another march, proceeding from Eaton Square to the Albert Hall. The Pageant of Women's Trades and Professions was organised as part of the International Woman's Suffrage Conference which included delegates from over twenty nationalities. The pageant consisted of 'voteless' professions carrying symbols of their work on the half an hour march.

London was the venue for the 1909 ICN Congress which was to turn into an unexpectedly emotional and fiery affair. The conference was well attended; Holland, Finland, Denmark, and Canada were admitted to membership and two Japanese nurses arrived chaperoned by two Japanese doctors. The President of the ICN, an Australian, was unable to attend and so Ethel Fenwick, as president of the National Association of the host country, welcomed the foreign delegates. In her address, Ethel spoke of the international aspect of nursing, a profession with no national borders. Outside of Britain, registration had already become law in New Zealand, the Cape Colony and Natal, and in ten of the United States. Among the delegates on the platform, at the opening session in the Great Hall of Church House Westminster, was Annie Goodrich, President of the American Nurses' Association. She asked Ethel Fenwick to accept honorary membership of their Association – the only foreign nurse to receive this honour.

Suddenly and unexpectedly, the proceedings of Congress were interrupted by Sidney Holland, chairman of the London Hospital and staunch ally of its Matron, Eva Luckes. He told the gathering that the conveners of the Congress did not represent English nursing or English hospitals. He then presented a manifesto against registration signed by sixty-seven matrons, all of whom were members of the Central Hospital Council for London. In spite of his spirited argument, the resolution for registration was carried unanimously. Later, another resolution was passed in favour of votes for women. This lively London Congress ended in a social whirl when King Edward VII invited the nurses to Windsor. Not to be outdone, the American Ambassador entertained 600 nurses to a reception.

After twenty years of campaigning, progress towards registration was slowly gathering support and momentum – but there was a lot of work still to be done.

Chapter 7

# Battles, Deaths, and Victories 1910–1919

The new Edwardian age was politically turbulent. In England and Wales, the numbers of people receiving poor relief had increased to 800,000, while 250,000 were reduced to living in the dreaded workhouses. One of the most important social changes was that of attitude. Victorians had once believed that poverty was due to lack of hard work or aspiration, but now a more compassionate and understanding mood was beginning to prevail.

Ethel still managed to find time for relaxation, staying for weeks in August and September at her sister Clara's home of Dunningwell in Cumberland. One of the regular visitors to Dunningwell was Ethel's younger brother Eric. He had found a career in the army in the Grenadier Guards and, as Captain Eric Edmond Moffat Davidson Manson, he served for a time under Colonel Augusts Henry Lane Fox Pitt Rivers, the famous ethnologist and archaeologist. Eric, known in the family somewhat disparagingly as the 'Capitaine', had married Blanche, a relative of that distinguished man, and had two daughters. As a younger brother of two very outspoken women, and with a strong-willed wife, Eric was not always held in the highest esteem by his bossy older sisters, although he spent long periods of time at Dunningwell, especially after he and his wife had separated.

Dr Bedford Fenwick was by then a very respected gynaecologist in Wimpole Street and counted the famous Lillie Langtry, as well as members of the royal family, amongst his patients. When, at an afternoon tea party at Dunningwell, he was expected to hand around cakes to the assembled guests, he was bitterly offended. He later stated that he 'refused to return to Dunningwell to be a mere footman to a lot of backwoodsman neighbours being patronised by his sister-in-law Clara'. He never went back to Dunningwell again.

Away from her concerns with nurse registration and committee work, Ethel continued to maintain an interest in antiques and she would later assert that Lord Dureen had offered her a partnership in an antique business, but commitments to nursing and to the issue of women's votes meant that this interest remained merely a hobby.

The year 1910 saw the death of many influential people, including the much-revered Florence Nightingale. Ethel Fenwick always regretted that Florence Nightingale had supported Eva Luckes in her opposition to registration. Although recognising Florence Nightingale as a pioneer of nurse training, Ethel believed that this opposition was due to the length of time between Florence's experience of hospital nursing and the development of the registration movement. It was only too easy to become out of touch when isolated from the daily physical demands and practicalities of work.

Jean Dunant, founder of the Red Cross, died in this same year. He had shared the first Nobel Peace Prize in 1901 and had always acknowledged the inspiration and influence of the example of Florence Nightingale in his life and work.

A woman with a totally different approach to illness, Mary Baker Eddy, who, in 1879, had founded the Christian Science Church, also died in 1910. Rejecting modern medicine, she had been a firm believer in the power of spiritual healing and in the illusory nature of disease. Pneumonia was responsible for the death of the 68-year-old King Edward VII in May.

A more personal and devastating loss to Ethel Fenwick in March 1910 was that of her close friend and much respected colleague, Isla Stewart. Isla had been appointed matron of St Bartholomew's following Ethel's departure and, working closely with Ethel, she had instigated many nursing reforms and had a major influence on nurse training.

Born in Dumfriesshire in 1855, Isla Stewart had been educated at home before beginning her nursing career as a probationer at

St Thomas's Hospital, London in 1879. She made rapid progress and in 1887 was appointed matron at St Bartholomew's Hospital when her friend Ethel Manson retired. Isla was one of the founder members of the Matrons' Council and President until her death. She was keenly interested in education and training of nurses, was a member of several nursing associations and, in 1907, assisted with training of French nurses. For this work she was awarded with a medal struck especially in her honour. Following deteriorating health, she died at the relatively young age of 53, with her dear friend Ethel at her side. She was buried in her hometown of Moffat and a bronze plaque to her memory was installed in the Church of St Bartholomew-the-Less.

Isla had been a tactful influence on Ethel; she was always prepared to talk and try to reach agreements with the other parties in the campaign for registration. This distressing loss of her friend meant that Ethel became more autocratic and, eventually, isolated. Having fought for so important a cause so hard and so long it was to prove almost impossible for her to stop fighting.

Halley's comet appeared, Captain Robert Falcon Scott set off for the South Pole, and the World's Fair opened in Brussels. Wife-poisoner Dr Hawley Crippen was the first person to be captured by the use of wireless telegraphy when he was arrested on the SS *Montrose* after he had poisoned, dismembered, and buried his wife in a cellar in London. His attempts to start a new life in Quebec were thwarted by the new science of radio communications and he was hanged a few months later.

Causing hardly any reaction or protests in the rest of the world, Japan annexed Korea. Rebellion raged in Mexico, the Boy Scout movement spread to the USA, and the passionate tango arrived in ballrooms. British dockers went on strike, to be joined later by the miners. The newly developed X-rays proved invaluable in an early case of a young boy in New York when a nail was detected in his lung. Using a new and daring technique, an incision was made in the boy's neck and a forceps removal of the nail was guided by the X-ray images.

The American health department released Typhoid Mary in 1910 on condition that she never accepted employment that involved the handling of food. Unfortunately, an overly optimistic assessment of her intelligence was made, and she was never able to grasp the concept of her contagious condition, as future events would prove.

Ethel and the family were shocked by the sudden death of her brother-in-law, Charles John Myers. A military man, following his Sandhurst training, he had served as a Lieutenant of the 39th Foot regiment in 1866, and had been stationed in Bermuda until 1869. He had retired just before the regiment was posted to India in 1870. He later served in the Royal Cumberland Militia and Lincolnshire regiment, retiring as honorary major in 1866. He collapsed and died suddenly during the Sunday service in Thwaites Church on 4 September 1910, aged 76. Ethel's sister Clara was devastated. Despite her dislike of physical intimacy and refusal to have children of her own, their marriage had been a comfortable and affectionate one. Her mother had died two years earlier and now the big house must have felt very empty at times. She continued to live at Dunningwell with her servants and, like Queen Victoria, wore black ever afterwards.

New tactics were required in the registration battle. After a delegation to the Prime Minister had failed to secure any guarantee of government support for registration, Ethel Fenwick invited interested organisations to meet and join together in a common cause. Representatives of the trained nurses' organisations held a meeting in 1910 to discuss the possibility of a joint Bill. Those joining were the British Medical Association, the Matrons' Council, the Society for the State Registration of Nurses, the Fever Nurses' Association, the Irish Nurses' Association, the Scottish Nurses' Association, and the Association for the Promotion of the Registration of Nurses in Scotland. They all agreed to the formation of the Central Committee of the State Registration of Nurses, with Mrs Fenwick as one of the joint honorary secretaries, and decided to draw up a joint Bill. This Bill incorporated the three principles which Ethel regarded as beyond compromise – a minimum standard of three years' training as the qualification for registration; a uniform curriculum and examination for all nurses; and the appointment of a central nursing council to govern the profession. After twenty-one years of campaigning in Britain, this committee, representing eight different nursing organisations, had at last produced a Bill for Registration.

These were dangerous times; revolutionaries in Europe were trying to raise funds to help their comrades in Latvia and Russia. In January 1911, having fled to London, a small group of anarchists injured and killed unarmed policemen when robbing a jeweller's shop. They became trapped inside a house in Sidney Street in the East End of London and more than 1,000 troops and armed police were involved in what became known as the Siege of Sidney Street. When the house began to burn down, the fire brigade were forbidden to intervene, on the orders of Home Secretary Winston Churchill. Only two charred bodies were recovered, the third anarchist apparently having escaped. Newsreel cameras had captured the events and by that evening West End cinemas were showing the drama just a few hours after it had ended. The age of instant communication was on the horizon.

The Festival of Empire opened at the Crystal Palace in May 1911, and a few days later George V and his visiting cousin, the Kaiser, officially reasserted their friendship.

Excitement at the prospect of nurses' registration proved to be premature. Each year between 1910 and 1913, a Bill for Registration was introduced in the House of Commons as a Private Member's Bill – but on each occasion it failed to get a hearing through lack of government support. Arguing that they could not ignore the opponents of registration, the government ignored the wishes of the nurses.

Ethel Fenwick was very well aware that as long as women did not have the vote, they lacked political power and that her battle was far from over. Ten thousand nurses were represented by the Central Committee, but the total number of nurses in the country was 70,000. Frustrated by this discrepancy, in her journal she scolded nurses for not taking an interest in their profession and its future. Her views on the value of publicity were very modern, although in her evidence to the select committee in 1905 she had been forced to admit that the *British Journal of Nursing* was read only by a small intellectual minority of nurses.

On 17 June 1911, International Women's Day spread from the USA to Europe and more than a million men and women took part in a commemorative march. Between 40,000 and 60,000 supporters of women's suffrage marched through London. All sorts of people, from sweatshop workers to collegians and titled women, took part. Some wore historical costume, including that of Boadicea, Queen Victoria, and Catherine of Aragon. Seven hundred women who had been jailed for the suffragette cause carried lances with banners in the suffragette colours of purple, green and white, and the rally ended with a meeting in the Albert Hall, presided over by Emmeline Pankhurst.

Ethel Fenwick had been elected President of the Society of Women Journalists from 1910–1911 and, in this role, she represented the Society at the Coronation of King George V. On 23 June 1911, Westminster Abbey was decorated with red tulips, white lilies, and blue delphiniums for the impressive ceremony. Preparations in the Abbey beforehand included the use of the new vacuum cleaner, a machine still in its early stages of development. It was a large, bright red object with a five horse-power piston engine which travelled on a horse-drawn cart and was accompanied by a team of operators in white drill suits.

In Parliament, Prime Minister Herbert Asquith flexed his political muscle and, with the backing of King George V, threatened to create enough peers to swamp all opposition, and so ensured the passing of the Parliamentary Act, giving supremacy to the House of Commons. Free school meals, old age pensions, and labour exchanges had been introduced in the previous few years. The Welfare State began to take shape, as Lloyd George's National Insurance Act provided unemployment benefits and hastened the end of the hated and harsh Poor Law. A national strike of railway men, dockers, and carters in 1911 brought cities like Manchester close to famine and, in London, nineteen out of every 1,000 inhabitants died during a heatwave.

While plague, flood, and famine devastated China, discontent and rebellion began to thrive there in spite of some constitutional reforms. In Britain, in October 1911, Winston Churchill was appointed First Lord of the Admiralty and the British navy was organised into a state of constant readiness. Meanwhile, the world's largest liner, the White Star *Olympic*, was able to carry 1,316 passengers and included Turkish baths amongst its facilities. Amundson reached the South Pole – but there was no word of the Scott party. In Germany, at the Lister Institute, groundbreaking research was being made by Casimir Funk into substances that he named vitamins.

Moray-born Ramsay MacDonald became leader of the Labour party – his birthplace just a few short miles from that of Ethel Fenwick. Throughout his career, he managed to keep close contact with his north-eastern roots, and was a frequent correspondent and, whenever possible, walking companion to the influential Scottish naturalist, Seton Gordon. Increasing pressures of work meant time out exploring and walking in the Highlands could give Ramsay MacDonald much needed relief from his mounting responsibilities. Even Seton Gordon's letters, describing as they did the wildlife and the countryside of his beloved Scotland, brought a breath of welcome fresh air into the politician's dusty London offices.

At Rockefeller Institute New York, Dr Francis Peyton Roos claimed to have discovered a virus that caused cancer. The brilliant researcher Marie Curie was awarded her second Nobel prize for her discovery of the elements of plutonium and radium. Her husband had been killed in a road accident five years previously and he was given a posthumous award at the ceremony.

At the fourth International Congress of Nurses assembly held in Cologne in 1912, Ethel Fenwick proposed that the ICN inaugurate an educational memorial in the name of Florence Nightingale. Her proposal was unanimously accepted, but due to the Great War, it was over twenty years before arrangements could be made. Ethel Fenwick was appointed chairman of the memorial committee in Britain but it was not possible for the Florence Nightingale International Foundation to be inaugurated until 1934.

By 1912, there were many areas of disruption throughout the world. The Manchu Dynasty, along with the boy emperor, was overthrown in China and a provincial republic was established. Tensions in the Balkans became more volatile before the inevitable explosion. Irish Loyalists pledged to fight against Home Rule and in April the unsinkable *Titanic* sank. A few days later, a total eclipse of the sun was seen in London. Czarevitch Alexei, the eight-year-old son of Czar Nicholas II, was diagnosed as suffering from haemophilia, a hereditary illness passed through his mother's line. Kaiser Wilhelm II launched the world's biggest ship, the 50,000-ton *Imperator*, which had crew of 1,000 and could carry 4,100 passengers. British battleships were recalled from the Mediterranean in order to counter the growing German presence in the North Sea.

At the Olympics in Stockholm, women were permitted to compete in tennis and swimming while suffragettes underwent the pain, degradation, and dangers of being force-fed in English prisons. When a French doctor announced he had found a cancer-causing microbe, others reserved judgement. Greeted with much excitement, the discovery of 'Piltdown man' was announced – the fact that it was a hoax was not to be discovered until 1953. Dr Alexis Carrel won the Nobel prize for medicine after developing methods for sewing blood vessels together and for keeping organs alive outside the body by perfusion with a nutrient-rich solution. The next goal, that of transplanting organs, was now in sight, albeit some time away.

At last, in 1913, the mysterious disappearance of Captain Scott was solved when his body was found on the Antarctic ice, 10 miles from his depot. Using ponies and just a few dogs, he had reached the South Pole in January 1912, only to find that the more practical Amundsen, having taken advice from experienced travellers, had beaten him by thirty-five days.

German naval and army powers continued to expand. As one country attempted peace, others became belligerent; the Balkans signed a peace treaty but there were riots in Dublin and the Unionists formed a volunteer army. The revolutionary and guerrilla leader, Pancho Villa, stormed through Mexico, and the Red Cross set up a hospital there for the wounded of both sides. The Geiger counter was invented by Hans Geiger, a German physicist who worked at Manchester investigating beta-ray activity. Life was becoming easier for some – electric irons, sewing machines, and vacuum cleaners were becoming available and the first assembly line was established in Michigan, allowing a car to be built in three hours to meet the unprecedented demand for the Model T Ford.

Many people were moved at the death of a remarkable American woman – 92-year-old Harriet Tubman. An illiterate field worker, she had helped fellow black slaves escape to freedom along the 'Underground Railroad' and had led 300 slaves to safety. During the Civil War, she had served as a cook, nurse, scout, and spy with the Union in South Carolina and was hailed as a true heroine.

The first sickness benefit in Britain was implemented in 1913; sickness benefit was 10/- a week, unemployment benefit was 7/- and maternity benefit was set at 30/- a week.

Still demanding the vote for women, suffragettes broke the windows of the Home Secretary's London office. In April, Emmeline Pankhurst was again jailed, this time for inciting the destruction of the home of the Chancellor of the Exchequer. After carrying out yet another a hunger strike as promised, Mrs Pankhurst was reluctantly released from jail. Another imprisoned suffragette, Mary Richardson, began a hunger strike but she had less influence or notoriety and was force-fed. In May, fifty-seven suffragettes were arrested for attempting to present a 'votes for women' petition to King George at Buckingham Palace. Amongst them was Mrs Pankhurst, looking frail and ill after her incarceration. As the first Chelsea Flower Show opened, public meetings by suffragettes were banned. More than 2,000 petitions for votes for women, with over a million names, had been presented to Parliament by that time.

There was nationwide shock at the death of an English graduate, a hunger striker previously imprisoned nine times and enduring force-feeding on seven occasions for her suffragette activities. Forty-year-old Emily Wilding Davison died from injuries received when she fell under the King's horse, Anmer, at the Derby in June 1913. Some people thought she had attempted to pin suffragette colours on the animal. Anmer and the jockey were both unhurt and ran again two weeks later at Royal Ascot. However, Emily Davison never regained consciousness and died from her severe injuries a few days later. Vast numbers of suffragettes attended her funeral, perceiving her to be a true martyr for the cause. Members of the National Union of Women's Suffrage Societies made a pilgrimage to her London funeral along six main routes covering the country from Carlisle to Cornwall. Her body was carried in an open carriage drawn by four black horses, followed by four vehicles laden with wreaths from all over the world. Ten bands played funeral music in the procession from Victoria to King's Cross station. She was laid to rest in the family vault at Morpeth.

Meanwhile, a London brain specialist attempted the impossible when he wasted valuable research time trying to analyse and rationalise women's relationship with clothes. By 1914, the last of the Carolina parakeets died in captivity after the species had suffered the double misfortune of producing ideal plumage for decorating ladies' hats, and a proclivity for eating farmers' fruit. The last passenger pigeon died in captivity the same year, an estimated 9 billion birds having been shot for fun and for pig feed. If not for the work of Scotty Phillips, as described in a previous chapter, the American buffalo would probably have suffered the same extinction in the cause of sportsmanship.

Around this time, Ethel found herself in more trouble than usual. An acrimonious dispute and some adverse comments about an opponent resulted in prosecution and, to avoid publicity, the Fenwicks were obliged to make a substantial settlement of £1,000 out of court. At a time when anti-German feeling was at its height, it was unwise to make libellous comments about a rival professional.

Ethel and her husband separated just before the outbreak of the First World War. These two strong characters had worked well together on behalf of the nurses' cause but had found it increasingly difficult to live amicably together. They remained in regular contact and no overt scandal was attached to their situation. Dr Bedford Fenwick continued to support his wife in her ambitions to reform nursing into an accredited profession.

Europe was a powder keg and countries armed themselves for war. Heavy expenditure on arms continued in Germany but, as war clouds gathered, high society danced on, the tango taking over from the more sedate foxtrot. Under the command of Colonel Younghusband, the British 'opened up' Tibet, making it safe for Chinese rule and British trade. Thanks to the conquest of Yellow Fever and malaria, the Panama Canal, which had been started in 1879, was finally opened to traffic in August 1914. Fifty miles long and varying between 100 and 300 yards wide, it required three locks for ships to negotiate in order to compensate for changes in elevation. While Cecil B. DeMille founded Hollywood, there was other uplifting news from America when the brassiere was patented by Mary Phelps Jacob.

George Soper, official of the New York City Department of Health, began looking for Typhoid Mary once again when more typhoid epidemics broke out at a sanatorium in Newfoundland, New Jersey, and at Sloane Maternity Hospital in Manhattan. He discovered that Mary had worked as a cook at both places. She was at last found and returned to the isolation centre where she remained until her death in 1938, there being no other way to ensure that she did not pass on the infection to which she herself was immune.

In March 1914, yet another attempt was made to introduce the Nurses' Registration Bill. Like its predecessors, it failed on its second reading.

On 28 June 1914, Archduke Franz Ferdinand, heir to the throne of Austro-Hungary, and his wife were assassinated by a Serbian nationalist and the world changed irrevocably. War broke out and the government passed a rule disallowing all Private Members' Bills for the duration of the war. This was the end of all attempts for women's suffrage and for nurses' registration. In a desperate attempt to take the heat out of the Irish situation, where civil war threatened, the cabinet advised the King to summon British and Irish party leaders to a conference at Buckingham Palace.

The realities of war came to Paris in August. General Joseph S. Gallieni was made Military Governor and, collecting every available motor car and taxicab in Paris, rushed 80,000 reserved troops to successfully counterattack the advancing Germans. In London, the Metropolitan police rounded up 300 Germans and detained them in the Olympia complex. All over the country, people were arrested on suspicion of spying and many homes were ransacked by the authorities. Being a fierce patriot, Ethel Fenwick believed in the righteousness of the British cause, and was fully in favour of interning all Germans in Britain.

The King granted an amnesty and, in consequence, all jailed suffragettes and strikers were released without condition and suffragettes agreed to immediately cease their campaigning for the duration of the war. A major enlistment campaign began and the first of the UK troops were sent to join the French in fighting the Germans and Austrians. From the west of Scotland, the Hebridean Outer Isles sent more men to the front per capita than any other area of the British Isles. In December, the first aerial combat took place over Southend when, having flown up the Thames, two German planes were chased by two British aircraft at 9,000 feet and at the amazing speed of 70mph. Londoners were ordered to dim their lights and the serious business of war began to affect the whole population. The Great War spread to the Far East, the Middle East, the South Pacific, and to Africa.

A seemingly insignificant but in fact a major development in medicine occurred with the first citrated blood transfusion, given in a Brussels hospital. Introduced by a Belgian surgeon, citrate prevented blood clotting when bottled. This development enabled countless lives to be saved with blood transfusions.

Ethel Fenwick was not alone in trying to break down barriers for causes she knew to be of long-term importance. Establishment prejudices appeared insurmountable, and enormous determination and persistence were required to fight and break these prejudices and inequalities. Dr Elsie Inglis had already fought long and hard to establish her place in medicine. By 1914, she was a much respected and very experienced doctor, and she offered her services and those of 100 female staff for the war effort. Her offer was totally rejected by the War Office and also rejected by the Red Cross.

Undeterred, and having raised money through a series of fund-raising speeches, Elsie Inglis organised a series of mobile hospitals to go into the field. A further offer to the War Office was again rejected and she was told to go home and sit still! She was 50 years old when the war began and in poor health, but she persisted. She offered her women's hospital to the French, who immediately accepted with gratitude. The first unit was established near Paris and was staffed entirely by women – doctors, nurses, orderlies, cooks, mechanics, and drivers. Within weeks, they had transformed a crumbling Cistercian Abbey into an efficient 100-bed hospital with operating theatre, dispensary, laboratory, and X-ray unit powered by its own generator. The team coped with ancient plumbing and bitter cold winters, and X-rays were often developed in a fish kettle. The number of beds doubled and a second unit was set up while they dealt with some of most gruesome casualties between 1915 and 1919.

In 1915, Dr Inglis also established another three medical units in Serbia, where they had to deal with typhoid as well as war wounded. During a retreat over the Serbian mountains, she was captured by the Austrians but, undaunted, she carried on working, looking after prisoners despite being one herself. Repatriated, she returned to help the Serbs in 1917, who were now fighting the Russians. She established yet another hospital in Odessa.

More than 1,000 women worked with the Scottish Women's Hospitals in the First World War and, of these, seventeen lost their lives. Dr Inglis was evacuated from Odessa by the navy in 1917 because of her worsening illness. She died, aged 53, the day after arriving in Newcastle. At her funeral, attended by several heads of state, she was given full military honours. She was decorated by France and Russia, but not by Britain, where the establishment still could not accept the non-domesticated woman. Elsie Inglis fought three wars: one against establishment male prejudice, one against the horrors of war, and the final one against the disease in her own body.

Ethel Fenwick had her own battles to fight during the war. Now in her late fifties, the world she had grown up in was gone forever. While there had been many changes and developments, improvements in her chosen field had not moved swiftly enough in spite of all her hard work. The government had delegated responsibility for organising the voluntary nursing services to the British Red Cross Society and this met with her vehement opposition. The National Council for Trained Nurses, with Ethel Fenwick as president, passed a resolution at its annual meeting in December 1914, placing on record its 'unqualified disapproval' of the manner and organisation of the nursing of sick and wounded soldiers in military and auxiliary hospitals at home and abroad. As she recorded in the *British Journal of Nursing* supplement of 30 January 1915, the resolution called upon the Secretary of State for War to prevent the expenditure of public subscriptions on 'inefficient nursing and the subjection of the sick and wounded to the dangerous interference of untrained and unskilled women'.

This was an attack on the members of the Voluntary Aid Detachments, and the amateur hospitals run by aristocratic ladies in their country houses whose well-intentioned voluntary but unskilled work had been encouraged by the BRCS. Trained nurses were disappointed that, after years of campaigning for statutory recognition of professional status, they still had to contend with government departments which regarded nursing as relatively unskilled, philanthropic work. When it became apparent, as early as spring of 1915, that there was a serious shortage of nurses, Ethel Fenwick did not hesitate to point out that had the registration of nurses been introduced the problem would not have occurred:

> Had the expert opinion of nurses themselves, expressed over and over again for the last quarter of a century, been heeded by the government the shortage would never have assumed the present serious dimensions ... They have pleaded for the passing of a Nurses Registration Act ... Such a Register would at the present moment be invaluable, both as the evidence of the qualifications of nurses seeking appointments, and as affording a means of communicating with trained nurses throughout the kingdom.
> (*British Journal of Nursing* editorial, 27 May 1915)

The first British air raid casualties occurred in Britain in January 1915, when a Zeppelin dropped bombs on King's Lynn and Great Yarmouth. In the distant Dardanelles, British troops fought their way ashore at Gallipoli to be quickly oppressed by heat, disease, and flies. They built trenches, which began to fill with dead and wounded in the struggle for Gallipoli, as the Turks mounted terrifying night attacks. In other bloody conflicts, Germans used gas at Ypres and Turks slaughtered thousands of Armenians. Captain Fergus Bowes-Lyon of the Black Watch, brother to the future Duchess of York, fell in action at Loos and an entire platoon of British troops were blinded by gas bombs.

Tragic casualties occurred in places other than the war zones – in 1915, en route to Liverpool to embark for Gallipoli, 215 men of 7 Battalion Royal Scots were killed in a train crash between Kirtlebridge and Gretna. A signalling error was responsible for the crash and derailment of the troop train and a local passenger train. The accident was compounded a few minutes later when the London to Glasgow express ploughed into the derailed trains and into the dazed and injured passengers. Mistaken for German prisoners of war, the shocked and dishevelled survivors were stoned by civilians. Rescuers were hindered by a fire which broke out when gas cylinders exploded. Following this disaster, steps were taken to ensure inflammable materials were stored apart from passenger areas in future. The loss of life in this accident remains the highest in British rail history.

New York held a great Easter parade; the *Lusitania* was sunk 10 miles off Ireland with the loss of 124 US lives, and Japan began squaring up to China over territorial, mineral, and fishing rights. Italy allied itself with Britain against Austria; and pacifists resigned from the US government when President Wilson prepared for war.

The Mayor of Chicago, concerned with more local issues, implemented restrictions on Sunday liquor sales. Henry Ford, along with 120 other pacifists, made a peace mission to Europe but had to call it off when he became ill. The mission had intended to help shorten the war – however, his strategy never took concrete form and he was ridiculed for his naiveté. Keir Hardie died of pneumonia, aggravated, it is said, by exhaustion and despair at the inability of unionism to prevent the war.

The Germans caused outrage when they executed Nurse Edith Cavell. In 1907, this nurse from Norfolk, who had trained at the London Hospital under Eva Luckes, had been appointed the first matron of the Berkendael Institute, Brussels, where she greatly improved the standard of nursing there. After the German occupation of Belgium, she became involved in an underground group formed to help British, French, and Belgian soldiers reach neutral territory. The soldiers were sheltered at the Berkendael Institute, which had become a Red Cross hospital, and about 200 men had been given aid. After letters of gratitude to her were intercepted, Cavell and several others were arrested in August 1915. They were brought before a court-martial and Edith Cavell was sentenced to death, despite the efforts of the US and Spanish ministers to secure a reprieve. Though legally justified, the execution of a nurse on a charge that did not include espionage caused great public indignation and disgust. Her martyrdom is said to have resulted in a 30 per cent increase in army recruitment. After the war, her body was brought back to her home city of Norwich for reburial and a statue of her was erected in central London.

Back in Britain, women were called to help the war effort by working in munitions factories. Many had never worked outside the home before but found themselves doing heavy and extremely dangerous jobs producing weapons. Believing that it would help increase arms production, King George V offered to give up alcohol in order to encourage armaments workers to abstain likewise.

The main goal of registration had still not been achieved but Ethel Fenwick characteristically threw herself wholeheartedly into everything she did. She was a member of the grand council and executive committee of the Territorial Force Nursing Service for the City and County of London, and a member of the ladies' committee of the Order of St John of Jerusalem. The experience and contacts she had made in other countries proved to be invaluable in her war efforts and she worked for the British Committee of the French Red Cross, which sent over 250 trained nurses to France to help the French nursing services.

Committee work was demanding, frustrating, and hard work, but past experience had given Ethel insight into what was most needed by nurses working in the field during a war situation. With her organisational skills, she and her colleagues were able to ensure the best was done for the nurses and, consequently, for the wounded. She was appointed honorary superintendent and treasurer of the French Flag Nursing Corps, under the French War Office, which involved selecting nurses for work in certain districts and visiting them periodically throughout France. She was later awarded the Médaille de la Reconnaissance française for her efforts and, after the war, was appointed by the committee to select nurses for work in the devastated areas of France.

Ethel and Dr Bedford Fenwick were living separate lives, and their only son Christian was fighting overseas, but they remained on polite terms. Dr Bedford Fenwick had set up another establishment at Cambridge Gate with a Miss Percy, but during the war he met Ethel amicably for lunch every month to discuss family business and support her nursing endeavours. Doubtless this arrangement gave the exhaustingly energetic Ethel more freedom to organise her activities and concentrate on the many committees she attended. The woman who had once been her son's nanny when Ethel had been busy with her campaigning was, by this time, Ethel's devoted housekeeper.

In March 1916, Ethel's brother, Captain Eric Edmund Moffat Manson, died aged 59. He had been known in the family as an affable kindly character who had no ambitions or experience other than that within the army. His headstone was inscribed 'A cheerful giver'.

War was a catalyst in encouraging nurses to do something about the disorganised state of their profession. At the end of 1915, the Matron-in-Chief of the British Red Cross Society, Sarah Swift, approached the Chairman of the British Red Cross Society, Arthur Stanley, who was a well-known 'neutral' on the issue of State Registration. Together they proposed the establishment of a College of Nursing, to promote a standard training for nurses. They invited the support of the matrons and hospital managers of the country's nurse training schools. After an encouraging response, the College of Nursing was launched as a limited company in April 1916.

The pro-registration lobby was divided in their response to the College of Nursing. By now, after her long years of struggle, Ethel Fenwick was very suspicious of any involvement of managers. Age had not moderated her temperament, and she was now without the restraining influence of her good friend Isla Stewart. When the College of Nursing was founded, many efforts were made to bring her in, but she was unable to accept its constitution and threw away one of her last opportunities to represent British nurses. Constant battling had dulled her ability to compromise and she thought the aims of the College were a distraction from the real cause of State Registration. However, some supporters of registration, such as the Matron of the General Hospital Birmingham, Ellen Musson, and the Matron of the Royal Free London, Rachel Cox-Davies, supported the College of Nursing. They believed that bringing the College behind the registration cause was better than leaving it open to the influence of its opponents.

Times were becoming more chaotic and men were fighting and dying for causes all over the world. Pursuing his own agenda in Mexico in January 1916, and unconcerned with the European War, Pancho Villa shot 18 US hostages in an attempt to involve the US in his own battle. In March, his troops were routed by a surprise attack led by Brigadier General John J. Pershing. In Europe, the longest and bloodiest battle of the war began in February, when the Germans attacked on a 25-mile front at Verdun. More than one million men were killed before Henri Petain achieved victory in June.

William Willet's daylight-saving plan was adopted in Britain and clocks were put forward one hour in summer. Britain was distracted by the Easter Rising of Irish Nationalists in Dublin, when Sir Roger Casement, leader of the Irish separatists, and his aides attempted to land an arms shipment for the use of the rebel groups. He was hanged as a traitor in June. That month, the British lost 6,907 men in the North Sea at the Battle of Jutland.

Life in London came to a shocked standstill at the news of the loss of Viscount Kitchener of Khartoum, of the Vaal, and of Aspall. Lord Kitchener, as he was generally known, was a British Field Marshal, Imperial administrator, conqueror of the Sudan, Commander-in-Chief during the South African War, and eventually the Secretary of State for War at the beginning of the First World War. He had been a ruthless and determined soldier and organised armies on a scale unprecedented in British history. The public idolised him, but his cabinet colleagues found his reluctance for delegation and for teamwork a problem, and in spite of being relieved of various responsibilities he had refused to step down. A German mine ended his career when the ship he was travelling on, the cruiser HMS *Hampshire*, was sunk off the Orkney coast on 5 June 1916.

July 1916 saw 60,000 British casualties on the Somme. A British secret agent, T. E. Lawrence, later to be revered as Lawrence of Arabia, was becoming embroiled in Arab affairs, which eventually led to him influencing the rebellion in the Arabian desert. By September, British tanks were being used for the first time on the Somme battlefields. A Squadron of German Zeppelins staged a bombing raid on the east coast of Britain, and one was brought down over London.

In America, President Wilson announced his support for votes for women to 4,000 delegates at the September suffrage gathering in New Jersey. Margaret Sanger, a public health nurse, who had studied in London, stated her belief that no social progress would be possible – especially where poverty existed – unless birth control was practised. She had previously been jailed for thirty days for opening a birth control clinic in Brooklyn, and was later indicted for sending birth control information through the US mail.

British and Greek ships were sunk by German submarines and a U-53 passed near the coast of Rhode Island, sinking more British and Norwegian ships. An outraged President Wilson ordered US destroyers to patrol the New England coast in search of German vessels. Jeanette Rankin, an exponent of women's rights and Montana republican, travelled the campaign trail on horseback and became the first Congresswoman ever elected to the US Congress. She believed her 25,000-vote victory was because 'the spirit of pioneer days was still alive'.

While the World War raged on, the US had the most prosperous year in its history. Ford produced even cheaper cars and made plans to double production. Wages rose and unemployment became almost non-existent as a record iron and steel output was achieved and many luxury goods were manufactured. Women were working in factories in America, but most labour unions refused to admit women. This resulted in women's health and pay being neglected, with 91 per cent of them earning less than men for equivalent work. Many employers considered that it would be the patriotic duty of women to leave their work and return to the kitchen sink and domestic duties once the men returned from the war.

Continuing with his research, Albert Einstein developed an extension of his theory of relativity but his fellow scientists were unable to test this new theory until the war ended.

It took some time before the British public began to appreciate the horrendous reality of the battles in the French trenches. Between February and July, the French repulsed a major German offensive at Verdun, with devastating losses on both sides. From July to November 1916, the battle of the Somme resulted in an appalling number of casualties and became a metaphor for futile and indiscriminate slaughter. In 1916, President Wilson declared that the world had the right to live in peace and called for a League of Nations to be set up when the war ended in order to prevent further wars.

Having suffered horrendous losses, the Allies retreated from Gallipoli in October and 90,000 remaining men were evacuated – thankfully without further loss. Having survived the horrors, flies, and diseases of Gallipoli, many were then sent on to face the muddy, bloody trenches of the Somme battlefields and the Western Front.

Increasing reliance was being placed on women workers in factories, women tram drivers, porters, railroad workers, and many other jobs previously thought of as men's work. After much debate and disagreement, conscription was belatedly introduced. Asquith, unable to get his cabinet to agree on the formation of a War Council, resigned as Prime Minister and was replaced by Lloyd George.

As the bloody year of 1916 ended, in Russia the monk Rasputin was assassinated by members of the Russian nobility who felt he held too much influence on their royal family. One of the assassins, Oxford educated Prince Felix Youssoupoff, was a friend and correspondent of the Scottish naturalist, Seton Gordon, himself in frequent correspondence with Ramsay MacDonald. Prince Youssoupoff and his wife, a niece of the Czar, were among the wealthy Russians who managed to get away to England on the HMS *Marlborough* before the chaos of the Revolution overtook the country. The Russian nation was starving, a situation worsened by bureaucratic ineptitude. Striking Russian workers demanding 'bread of freedom' were gunned down by Czarist troops. After months of turmoil and heavy losses on the German front, the Czar abdicated with the words 'May God help Russia'.

In April 1917, the US finally entered the war, with President Wilson weeping at the prospect of sending so many young men to their deaths. The Greek King Constantine was forced to abdicate in favour of his second son. As the brother-in-law of the Kaiser, he had violated Greek neutrality in different ways, including permitting German ships to use Greek bases. In July, the British royal family adopted the name House of Windsor, deeming it more acceptable than continuing to call themselves by the Germanic name of the House of Saxe-Coburg-Gotha. By this time, the war was costing Britain £7 million daily. In Russia, by August, the Czar and his family had been moved out of their palace and held captive by Bolshevik forces. Within a few months, the Bolsheviks seized power in a virtually bloodless coup.

Prejudice and injustice persisted regardless of other serious world conflicts. Seventeen people died as a result of a riot in Texas when a regiment of black troops were quartered in Houston. The trouble started after a soldier, objecting to a white policeman slapping a black woman, was beaten and sent to jail.

Supplies of Turkish tobacco were disrupted by the war and British troops were bogged down in Flanders mud. In October, the notorious Mata Hari was shot at dawn after being found guilty of espionage. Contrary to the legend of her being a beautiful, exotic, and intelligent spy, the true story is a pathetic and sordid tale of a somewhat naïve woman. She was one of at least a dozen female spies executed by France in the Great War.

The British government supported Zionist aspirations of establishing a permanent homeland for Jewish people in Palestine. Helped by the efforts of T. E. Lawrence, who organised the dynamiting of railroads and bridges, General Allenby claimed Jerusalem as British territory. The actions of 'Lawrence of Arabia' captured the public imagination at a time when tales of successful escapades and heroism were badly needed to keep up morale.

Following the disintegration of the Imperialist forces during the Bolshevik Revolution, 1918 saw the creation of the Red Army in Russia, founded by Leon Trotsky. While Russia was torn by civil war, sixty German planes bombed Paris in a night raid, killing 106 civilians.

The German flying ace Manfred von Richthofen, known as the Red Baron, was shot down and killed at the Somme in April 1918. He had destroyed eighty Allied planes in less than two years. Paris was pounded by 'Big Bertha', a massive howitzer which was moved around on railroad cars. 'Bertha' killed over 800 people and was the last of its kind. In July 1918, the Czar and his young family were all brutally executed, so ending three centuries of rule by the Romanov dynasty.

In spite of the war, many people continued to concentrate their energies on other more long-term issues. In 1918, British paleobotanist and author Marie Stopes, BSc, DSc (who was married to Humphrey Verdon Roe, co-founder of the burgeoning A. V. Roe aircraft firm), caused controversy with her books *Married Love* and *Wise Parenthood*. This was the first time birth control had been discussed in a publicly available book and it caused great shock and outrage, with the books being banned in America. Previous proponents of birth control had seen it as a method for controlling overpopulation and consequent poverty. Marie Stopes caused controversy mainly because she perceived birth control as a means of enhancing marriage relationships and as a way to save women from the physical strain of excessive childbearing.

When the First World War began, the women's suffrage organisations had diverted their energy into the war effort. Their dedication and patriotic work did much to win the public to the suffragist cause. The need for the enfranchisement of women was finally recognised, and the resulting Representation of the People Act was passed by the House of Commons in June 1917 and by the House of Lords in February 1918. From then on, all men over 21 and, for the first time, women aged 30 or over could vote. Shortly afterwards, another act was passed enabling women to sit in the House of Commons and, in December 1918, women voted for the first time in a General Election.

By July 1918, the Allies had begun to start to push the Germans back. Recently developed anti-tetanus vaccinations were used on the troops but suddenly a new disease occurred which cut a swathe through the civilian population as well as the fighting men. An outbreak of a virulent influenza epidemic killed millions of people worldwide. The first major outbreak appeared in Spain, and from Europe, moved on to Asia. The epidemic spread rapidly through overcrowded armies and malnourished civilian populations who were already weakened by war. Many people felt as if the end of the world was upon them.

At long last, the 'war to end all wars' was over. At 5.00 am on 11 November 1918, the Armistice document was signed in Foch's railway carriage at Rethondes. At 11.00 am that day, the First World War came to an end. Communications were not instantaneous in those days and it was only after all parties involved had been notified and the event coordinated satisfactorily that, at 11.00 am on 15 November 1918, peace was officially and finally declared. Britain suffered over 750,000 war casualties, many of them in trench warfare at the Western Front in France. Loss of these lives and of their influence on future generations would result in the development of a very different nation.

Peace was celebrated with unprecedented public rejoicing. As the Armistice took effect at 11.00 am, fireworks, which had previously been used as warnings of impending disaster, were fired throughout the country. People rushed into the streets, cheering and waving flags, hoisting servicemen shoulder-high, and dancing cakewalks until the early hours. After four years of silence, when Big Ben struck one o'clock, London was ablaze with flags flying from thousands of rooftops. King George V and Queen Mary drove to the centre of London to Hyde Park though huge crowds and thousands packed Downing Street to cheer the Prime Minister Lloyd George and members of the coalition cabinet. Streetlights were once again ablaze and blackout curtains were torn down. Licensing laws were ignored as pubs were packed until they ran out of beer. Sadly, such public gatherings provided ideal conditions for further transmission of the burgeoning deadly influenza virus.

Despite the war, momentum for change within nursing had not been lost. The College of Nursing had gained wide support among matrons, who encouraged their staff to join the organisation. By 1918, the College had a membership of 8,000 and, in response to its members, drew up a Bill for the Registration of Nurses. Negotiations were held with the Central Committee for the State Registration of Nurses in an effort to produce a joint Bill, but after many months, agreement proved impossible. Both parties published separate bills, and Ethel Fenwick denounced the College Bill as an 'employers' bill' because it failed to give nurses the degree of self-government which she regarded as essential for professional independence. The profession and the nursing press were divided in their support for the two bills, and both groups lobbied their MPs separately.

While the post-war peace proposals were being worked out, the League of Nations charter was adopted at Versailles in February 1919. This was the year that Theodore Roosevelt died suddenly in his sleep. Famous for his pronouncement that the proper way to conduct foreign affairs was to 'speak softly and carry a big stick', he had been awarded the Nobel Peace Prize in 1906 for mediating the end of the Russo-Japanese War.

In February 1919, Eva Luckes died. Born in 1854, she had been matron of the London Hospital for thirty-nine years and had always been a fierce opponent of Ethel and her ideas of nurse registration. Matron Luckes had been suffering from ill health, arthritis, diabetes, cataracts, and impaired mobility and, when she became acutely ill, she was nursed by Sisters from her hospital. Over the years, she had written passionately about her belief in the qualities essential in a good nurse: 'There are many belonging to us of whom we can say with just pride "They help all with whom they come into contact – not because they can produce any number of Certificates but because they love so much!"' She had also written: 'if a Nurse is to be worthy of her calling, her work must be inspired by the right spirit of Nursing – i.e. of active sympathy with suffering manifested by unwearied kindness and unselfish devotion to those entrusted to her care'. Despite heavy criticism and her fierce objection to registration, Eva Luckes had many successes. Nurses who had been under her training worked all over the world, including Nurse Edith Cavell. In recognition of her work over the years, Eva Luckes had been awarded the Commander of the Order of the British Empire, Royal Red Cross, and Lady of Grace of the Order of St John of Jerusalem in England.

At last progress was being made in nursing, in spite of two factions, the group formed by Ethel (the Central Committee for the State Registration of Nurses) and the College of Nursing, both lobbying for their own different approaches to registration. Early in 1919, the Bill of the Central Committee for Registration had been introduced to Parliament. This Bill survived its first reading in the Commons and, in the interests of the profession, the College of Nursing decided to support it on the second reading. At the committee stage, however, the College promoted several amendments which it considered essential to make the Bill acceptable. There were so many amendments that the College withdrew its support and promoted its own Bill in the House of Lords. One can only imagine the determination, arguments, impassioned speeches, and dogmatic discussions that went on between all the individuals involved.

The College Bill had survived its first reading in the Lords in May 1919 and was waiting for second reading when the Minister of Health, Dr Addison, asked both parties to withdraw their individual bills on the promise that the government would introduce a Bill for the Registration of Nurses as soon as possible.

In Italy, the son of a blacksmith and a schoolteacher, Benito Mussolini, founded his own party and published his fascist manifesto. Among the demands in the manifesto were universal suffrage, the right of women to vote, autonomy for local governments, an end to secret diplomacy, the confiscation of church property, the creation of a purely defensive army, an eight-hour working day, a minimum wage, and retirement at the age of 55. It all appeared so very reasonable.

Peace was not universally sought; border clashes between the British and Afghans brought the frontier up in arms. The Treaty of Versailles was signed in June 1919, finally ending the war, but the Germans scuttled seventy-four of their captured ships at Scapa Flow, Orkney, rather than surrender them. This act of defiant despair was watched by horrified Orkney schoolchildren as fifty-two of the ships sank into the cold, dark waters of the Flow.

The end of war saw a resumption of serious and daring Paris fashions. Outrageously, some outfits were designed to be worn with no corsets, allowing women the freedom to move and breathe naturally. At last, there was no need for extreme lacing-in of waists in order to attain the perfect hourglass shape. The war had accelerated the freedom of physical movement for women and the swooning, languishing, and internal disorders frequently caused by tight corsets was no longer considered fashionable or desirable. Paris had now also discarded tailor-made mannish designs; soft materials were used, skirts were being worn a bold 7–8" from the ground, while glamorous, backless evening gowns became desirable and acceptable.

Having reached the age of 60, Ethel enjoyed old age from then on, saying frequently, 'I am a very old lady and I must be respected', and instead of her previous bright colours, she took to wearing black and grey, proclaiming her belief in wholesome food, and plenty of sleep. She had become a grandmother and treated her two grandchildren with benign affection.

She always carried a long umbrella with a tassel and had a habit of poking things with it. On her regular summer holidays in Cumberland, she would walk in her highly polished black shoes, poking about in country lanes, breathing deeply for the good of her health. The regular family gatherings at Dunningwell continued during August and September, when she travelled north to spend time relaxing away from the demands of London life. High standards of behaviour were maintained, and there were inevitable clashes of personality between strong-minded family members.

Alcock and Brown made the first non-stop flight across the Atlantic in June 1919 and, after experimenting with rockets since 1909, Professor

R. A. Goddard of Massachusetts announced that a trip to the moon would eventually be possible. This ludicrous statement caused him to be ridiculed by the press. He wasn't the only scientist to bemuse ordinary mortals with his prescience. In December 1919, an eclipse was to prove the validity of Einstein's theory of relativity, which he had announced in Berlin in 1915. Only a few of the world's intellectuals understood his complex calculations.

Race riots in Chicago in July resulted in thirty-one dead and 5,000 injured before military troops succeeded in quelling the chaos. The influenza pandemic continued to race around the world with unprecedented speed, spreading rapidly through armies and striking swiftly at the civilian populations that were already weakened by the effects of stress and poor diet. Deaths among civilians exceeded those amongst the troops and more servicemen died from influenza than died in battle. Causing millions of deaths in China, it was estimated that over 20 million people died worldwide as casualties of the deadly virus.

In December 1919, Lady Astor made history when, as the Tory candidate for Plymouth, she was the first female Member of Parliament to take her seat in the House of Commons. Known for her liveliness and wit, she remained as an MP until 1945 and, as well as questions relating exclusively to women, she concentrated mainly on educational and social problems.

The nursing battle was slowly reaching its finale. When Parliament reassembled in the autumn, the Government Bill for the Registration of Nurses was introduced, passed, and became law on 23 December 1919. Ethel Fenwick watched what she described as the last act in the drama from the public gallery. After years of determined hard work, the idea that had germinated long before she founded the Society for the State Registration of Nurses in 1902 had come to fruition.

The St Bartholomew's Hospital journal recorded proudly:

Barts has played a big part in securing the State Registration of Nurses.

1) a former matron (Mrs. Bedford Fenwick) initiated the reform:
2) a one-time Professor of Anatomy, a Minister of Health (Dr. Addison) introduced the Bill and placed the Nursing Acts on the Stature Book and 3) the Treasurer of the Hospital (Lord Stanley) carried them through the House of Lords.

From its early military and religious heritage, nursing had come of age and, with its disciplined, accredited training, had finally been recognised as a skilled and respected profession.

Chapter 8

# Registration and Professionalism 1919–1946

...ed for the establishment
...be responsible for the
...s. The Council was to
...ster. While registration
...sible for details of that
...of Health, Dr Addison.
...Provisional Council and

...on 10 January 1920:

...e of the managers of
...ll reform by state aid
...blic spirit exhibited by
...at time. Had hospital
...a sense of public and
...ssion of nursing would
...and well-renumerated
...although the act lays
...e whole superstructure
...).

The country was shocked by the dreadful murder in January 1920 of 54-year-old Florence Nightingale Shore – goddaughter of her famous namesake. Florence Shore had recently been demobilised from the Queen Alexandra's Nursing Corps after service in France and had been decorated for her war work. Like Ethel, Florence had been educated at

Middlethorpe Hall school. Her battered body was discovered on board the London to Brighton train and her murderer was never caught.

The first meeting of the League of Nations, consisting of France, Britain, Italy, Japan, Belgium, Spain, Brazil, and Greece, took place in February 1920 but, with the clarity of hindsight, it is possible to see the seeds of future trouble being sown.

Prohibition took effect in the United States of America as beer, wine and liquor were banned, unwittingly allowing the growth of crime and corruption. There were race riots in Chicago in July, which were quelled by military troops and resulted in thirty-one dead and 500 injured. In Germany a monarchist coup failed to restore the monarchy. Adolph Hitler, propaganda chief of the German Workers Party, announced his goals, which included anti-Semitism and anti-capitalism. French troops occupied the Ruhr as German troops mobilised to fight a communist army, the French believing that German military action was a violation of the Versailles treaty.

In the world of fashion, hemlines rose up to the knee and the age of the rebellious and outrageous 'flappers' began. By August 1920, after more than eighty years of trying, women in America at last won the right to vote – many years later than the women of Australia (1902) and New Zealand (1893). In October 1920, the first 100 women were admitted to Oxford to study for degrees.

Turmoil continued in Mexico while, in the streets of Belfast, Irish rioters protested against the severe restrictions of British rule. Tensions worsened when fourteen British officers and officials were killed in Dublin at the start of a day of violence. Reinforcements were swiftly sent and 43,000 soldiers joined the special constabulary, known as the Black and Tans. Violence escalated, order was restored by troops in armoured cars and 21 November 1920 was later known there as Bloody Sunday. The Lord Mayor of Cork died in Brixton prison after a seventy-four-day hunger strike and by December the British had partitioned Ireland.

By 1921, the serious issue of short skirts was causing anxiety and outrage, and police in Pennsylvania were required to enforce women to wear skirts no less than 4" below the knee. The new film industry was burgeoning and Rudolph Valentino, in the film *The Sheik*, had audiences swooning. The new popular bobbed haircut was a much safer style for women working in factories but was not approved of by traditionalists. Women wearing make-up met with disapproval, and smoking and drinking had to be indulged by women in private. Queen Mary became the first woman to be awarded an Oxford degree, and the first Stopes birth control clinic was opened in the Holloway district of London. Kitty MacCurran became the first woman to be killed by Sinn Féin in Ireland when she was taken from her home, accused of being an informer and shot.

Regardless of their excellent results in medical school, nearly all hospitals still refused to take female medical students. A seemingly small but very significant development was made when a cotton mill employee made a ready-to-use bandage for his new bride, who was constantly cutting herself when working in the kitchen. His 'Band Aid' was to become an indispensable item in every first aid kit from homes to hospitals and workplaces.

America donated aid as Europe was hit by hunger and unemployment, but the issue of short skirts continued to occupy disproportionate attention there and legislation was brought in to keep hemlines from rising more than 3" above the ground. New styles of dance and dress swept the nation and were decried as an offence against decency.

As the United States became swamped by emigrants from war-torn Europe, immigration restrictions were introduced. Race riots in Tulsa, Oklahoma erupted in May 1921 following the accusation of rape made against a black American, a 19-year-old bootblack who had simply but accidentally stumbled against a white teenage girl. The situation was inflamed by the editor of the *Tulsa Tribune* exhorting readers to 'Lynch a nigger tonight'. The Scottish pastor of the First Presbyterian Church, the Reverend Charles Kerr, managed to calm the situation for a while until the editorial exhortation took effect. As black Americans had been successfully competing for jobs in the district, tension was already present and there was a distinct danger that there would be a lynching. By the time peace had been restored, over 11,000 houses had been burnt as well as twenty-three churches, a public library, and many business premises. It is estimated that over 300 people were killed, including a baby which was shot while lying in its crib. There was no re-housing policy and 1,000 black Americans spent the winter in tents. Pains were taken to hush up the riots that had taken place in 'the land of the free', and to hide the fact that 6,000 white supremist men had joined the Ku Klux Klan.

Mussolini made himself 'Il Duce' and leader of the National Fascist Party in Italy. Starvation and cholera swept through Russia. The communist party was formed in China and library assistant and primary school teacher, Mao Tse-tung, attended its first congress.

Many new medicines were being developed. Cocaine and heroin flooded into America, having been smuggled from Germany through South America. Germany had developed synthetic drugs like Novocain, aminol, and veronal, when war had cut off normal supplies.

In July 1921, a life-changing and life-saving medicine was created when insulin was isolated from a dog's pancreas by a 29-year-old Canadian, Dr G. F. Banting, and his student Charles Best, at the University of Toronto. Within a few months, it became widely available and changed the terminal prognosis of diabetes. Dr Banting was awarded the 1922 Nobel prize for his work.

In June 1921, the first premises of the General Nursing Council at 12 York Gate, London were opened by Princess Christian. On behalf of the Royal British Nurses' Association, Ethel presented her old friend and comrade-in-arms with a bouquet. The chairman of the council, Dr Priestly, addressing the Princess in his speech, said:

> You see around you not only the present members of the Council, but many who have fought the battle of Registration from its earliest days, and borne the heat and burden of a prolonged engagement, sometimes rebuffed but never discouraged, always persevering towards the goal they set out to win.

The register of nurses was opened on 30 September 1921. Qualified nurses had to pay a fee and existing nurses had until 1923 to be on the register. Having reverted to her original middle name, Ethel Gordon Fenwick was recorded as State Registered Nurse No. 1. After her long struggle, she certainly deserved the distinction of being recognised as Britain's first State Registered Nurse.

Remembering how long and how hard she had battled to achieve her objective, and how bitter was that battle over the years, it is understandable that a strong character like Ethel would be reluctant to trust others to set her project on the right tracks and ensure its integrity. As Chairman of the Registration Committee, Ethel Fenwick regarded herself personally responsible for the veracity of the qualifications of every nurse whose name was admitted to the register.

However, within the General Nursing Council, the process of registration was so slow that in December 1921 two-thirds of the council, including the chairman, resigned in protest. The Minister of Health intervened and asked Mrs Fenwick to resign from the committee – a request she firmly refused. Devious political manoeuvres were necessary. After several weeks, the Minister appointed a new chairman of the council and reinstated the councillors who had resigned. The council then passed a resolution, with immediate effect, that committees would be appointed on an annual basis. A new registration committee was appointed and Ethel Fenwick was humiliatingly excluded. She fought back through the pages of her journal – bitterly reproaching nurses for having allowed their professional independence to be compromised by College of Nursing.

> Had the majority of nurses taken an intelligent interest in their own affairs, acquainted themselves with the privileges granted to them by parliament ... acted for themselves, instead of allowing themselves to be manipulated by a company of lay men, there would have been a very different tale to tell.
>
> (*British Journal of Nursing* editorial, December 1922)

Ethel regarded the Registration Act as a great step forward, comparable to the enfranchisement of women, and the fact that nurses were given a two-thirds majority on the Council she claimed as a personal achievement. However, when the whole Council had been appointed, Ethel Fenwick and her supporters were in the minority among other nurse members, outnumbered by supporters of the College of Nursing. The proceedings of the first General Nursing Council were dominated by old animosities and it was inevitable the two factions would have trouble reaching mutually acceptable decisions.

The Nurses Act of 1919 had been accepted by Ethel as the long-awaited legislation on state registration and she was prepared to work within the terms of the Act as she saw them. However, her ideas on the role of the GNC were not shared by the majority of the Council members and, instead of compromising, she cut herself off from the representative body which she had worked for so long to establish. The *Nursing Times* commented on 8 April 1922: 'The nursing profession has suffered much from those whose public spiritedness has a strong flavour of personal antagonism to other leaders in the same good cause.'

The first election of councillors to the General Nursing Council took place at the end of 1922, but due to an administrative error, elections had to be held again in February 1923. It is not difficult to imagine the frustrations and disappointment this must have engendered. By then approximately 12,000 nurses were on the register and eligible to vote. The College of Nursing put up its own candidates, Ethel Fenwick and her supporters standing as independents to represent 'the free nurses' organisations'.

Mrs Fenwick lost her seat, and in a series of articles in her journal gave her frank and full views on the election under the title 'How the College Caucus Captured the Council'. Although now excluded from the General Nursing Council, she followed all its proceedings closely and reported all the decisions which affected the development of the profession. She criticised much, especially the failure to make the training syllabus compulsory and the lack of progress on the examination syllabus.

While Ethel Fenwick grew older, improving communications meant the world was growing smaller. In 1922, the first BBC national broadcast was made and the popular *Reader's Digest* magazine was set up. Although she was only 54, American reporter, Elizabeth Cochrane Seaman, known as Nellie Bly, died of pneumonia. She had become a famous traveller, managing the fastest solo trip around the world, but she preferred working on her crusades for social reform. In 1887, she had feigned insanity in order to investigate conditions at an asylum and her exposure of neglect and violence towards the inmates had resulted in nationwide reform.

The Ottoman Empire finally ended in Turkey and, due to a common public terror of communism, Mussolini was able to assume dictatorship in a bloodless takeover in Italy. The war had demanded a massive financial as well as personnel cost. In Britain, there were very few jobs for returning servicemen. Lloyd George's coalition government fell. Working from Einstein's quantum theory, Neils Bohr was awarded the Nobel prize for physics after managing to explain the internal structure of the atom.

The future President of the United States, Franklin Delano Roosevelt, contracted polio after swimming in Fundy Bay. Within two days, the 39-year-old was paralysed from the waist down. Perhaps as a reaction against the many sudden advances in medicine, Emile Coue propounded a new theory in 1923 – that of 'positive thinking'. He advocated the benefits of saying 'every day in every way I'm getting better' and so developing the mastery of will through the power of auto suggestion. However, his new theory would have been of no use in dealing with the 300 cases of smallpox that broke out in Scutari where, at long last, a treaty had ended the Greek-Turkish war. The Turks were keeping 10,000 Greek refugees in squalor at Scutari as they awaited deportation back to Greece. Positive thinking would not have helped Lord Carnarvon who, shortly after the discovery of the spectacular Tutankhamun's tomb in Egypt, died from blood poisoning following an insect bite acquired when opening the tomb.

The first Nazi party congress was held in Munich in 1923 and, during it, the treaty of Versailles was rejected as being too harsh. It was claimed that the French and Belgium occupation of the industrial region of the Ruhr destroyed the economy, causing German miners to cut production and thousands of people to be displaced from the Ruhr. Soon it was claimed to be cheaper to a light fire with German currency than to buy firewood and understandably this resulted in massive resentment, poverty, and unrest.

When Albert, Duke of York, married Elizabeth Bowes-Lyon in Westminster Abbey in April 1923, he was blissfully unaware of the monarchical role that awaited him. Great advances were being made in nutritional research thanks to the efforts of John Boyd Orr who had, in 1923, established the Rowatt Research Institute in Aberdeenshire. Providing proof of the nutritional value of milk, he was responsible for the introduction of free school milk for children in 1924. His argument for a national food policy, which took into account social needs, proved too revolutionary, but his future work was to prove invaluable.

In the United States, poverty encouraged people to compete in dance marathons. The desperate participants staggered around the dance floors for hours, hoping to win money prizes, but instead many of them only gained severely swollen ankles and experienced sudden and dramatic weight loss. Oklahoma was placed under martial law when the Ku Klux Klan, which claimed to have 1 million members, was outlawed. Meanwhile, having helped develop the life-saving gas mask, a black American, Garret Morgan, was busy developing modern life-saving traffic lights.

It was a sad time for Ethel Fenwick when her great friend Helena, Princess Christian of Schleswig-Holstein, died in June 1923, aged 77. The two had worked long and hard together for the benefit of nursing and, in recognition of their friendship, in 1888 Ethel had named her only son Christian.

By 1924, there was a financial boom and a foe of the Ku Klux Klan, America's first woman governor, democrat 'Ma' Miriam Ferguson, was elected in Texas. The man from Moray, Ramsay MacDonald, headed the first British Labour government. Greece became a republic and, in Turkey, Kemal Atatürk tried to introduce modernisation.

In spite of the many advances, medicine was not infallible even for the rich and influential. Doctors were unable to provide a cure for the son of Calvin Coolidge, 30th President of the USA, who, after cutting his foot playing tennis, died from septicaemia. The Nobel prize for medicine went to Dutchman William Einthoven, who had invented the electrocardiogram in the early 1900s then simplified it and enabled it to be manufactured with relative ease.

During the 1920s and 1930s, Ethel Fenwick continued to edit and write for the *British Journal of Nursing* but in 1924, due to falling readership, it changed from a weekly to a monthly publication. Ethel assumed that her readers were intelligent and professional and refused to alter her style in order to increase sales. Her *Journal* reported on the social and professional activities of nurses as well as the proceedings of various nursing organisations, whether in sympathy with her views or not. It also reported the ups and downs of the suffrage campaign – Ethel Fenwick regarding the vote as a right for professional women. She constantly urged nurses to take an interest in the issue and keep themselves informed of the facts.

The 1925 Matrimonial Clauses Act allowed, for the first time, women to divorce adulterous husbands. In spite of fears that this freedom for females would lead to an increase in divorce rates, many simply could not afford it. Women's pay was around half that of men and was not sufficient to support a family.

The old Central Committee for Registration of Nurses was renamed and became the Registered Nurses' Parliamentary Council. Through this Council, Ethel Fenwick was able to lobby MPs for intervention in what she considered the shortcomings of the General Nursing Council. She achieved her objective when eventually, in 1925, a Select Committee was appointed to consider certain aspects of the rules of the General Nursing Council.

The first congress of the ICN after the Great War was held in Helsinki in 1925. Ethel Fenwick had intended to go, always being a welcome guest at these social and professional functions. However, she remained in London to give evidence to the Select Committee on the GNC. A paper she had prepared for the Helsinki Congress, 'The trained nurse's Part in Peace', was read for her by a colleague at the Congress.

The Select Committee sat for less than six weeks and heard many witnesses including Ethel Fenwick. In its report the committee did not accept her point that the 1919 Nurses Act had intended that the training syllabus be compulsory. However, it did agree that the rule stipulating that six of the eleven representatives of the nurses on the general council should be matrons was contrary to the spirit of the Act, and that all eleven seats should be open to general trained nurses.

By this time wild swings were taking place on the Stock Exchange in Wall Street. Chiang Kai-shek became Chairman of the Chinese Republic and Hirohito was crowned Emperor of Japan. The new pastime of crossword puzzles became the latest craze. Joseph Shanks, president of United Artists, announced his belief that in the cinema, 'talkies' would prove to be just a temporary fad. In the United States, despite constant police raids on 'speakeasies' and a clamp down on the sale of alcohol, undiluted illicit alcohol had killed hundreds of people.

In London in July 1925, at Guy's Hospital, six-year-old Patricia Cheeseman was the first person to be successfully treated with insulin. A high school teacher in Tennessee, John T. Scopes, was indicted in 1925 under the state law for the crime of teaching the theory of evolution. This trial aroused furious debate between the proponents of the theory of evolution and the believers in a precise theory of creation as outlined in the Bible. By August, in America, the Ku Klux Klan was able to mount a parade of 40,000 members.

A significant difference in the lives of many women occurred when modern bikes were designed with dropped crossbars. This improvement meant that, at a time when it was unacceptable for them to wear trousers, women no longer offended sensibilities and could travel in a less ungainly and more modest manner.

Hindenburg was elected German president in April 1925 and the rise of the Nazi party in Germany was spurred by the desperation of millions of unemployed citizens. Following the war, the European unemployment figures had reached historic levels and worldwide economic depression deepened. The manual for the National Socialist Party, *Mein Kampf*, was published in July 1925.

France and Germany finally made peace with the Treaty of Locarno, Switzerland, in 1925, which resulted in the American Vice-President, Charles Dawes, sharing the Nobel peace prize with Neville Chamberlain for achieving this settlement.

In 1926, John Logie Baird demonstrated his new invention – the television. The first traffic lights in Britain were installed at Piccadilly Circus in London. In April 1926, a daughter, Elizabeth, was born to the Duke and Duchess of York, her destiny as future Queen unrecognised. The first general strike in British history began on 3 May 1926 and lasted for twelve days. It had been called in support of the miners, who had been protesting about pay cuts and longer hours. The miners continued their strike for a further six months, but eventually had to concede and their working day was increased from seven to eight hours.

The death of the film star Rudolph Valentino, at the age of 31 in August 1926, from a ruptured appendix and gastric ulcer, caused an outpouring of grief and one distraught fan shot herself. The escapologist Houdini died of peritonitis aged 52 in October 1926 following a blow to his abdomen. Medicine had not yet advanced sufficiently to enable a better outcome for such conditions.

Ethel and her family continued to spend their summer holidays at Dunningwell, where widowed Clara, who was devoted to dogs, nurtured a dog's graveyard with its several small inscribed headstones. Now married, Ethel's son Christian was living in Newcastle and the family entourage, complete with caged birds, dogs, goldfish, budgerigars, and maids would descend on Dunningwell to meet up for the annual gathering, which Clara called 'the invasion'. Children and their nanny were accommodated on the top floor in the fully equipped nursery, which lay empty the rest of the time as Clara had no children of her own.

Years later, Ethel's grandson David fondly recalled his time spent at Dunningwell. He remembered his aunt Clara was always dressed in increasingly fading black widow's attire. Regardless of her given name, the cook at Dunningwell was always known as 'Mary Cook' and the maids were always known as 'Margaret'. He heard whispers about one 'disgraced' maid and a dismissed gardener but never fully understood the rumours at the time. Clara would always leave the house through the conservatory so she could walk past the pet cemetery and on the anniversary of a pet's death she would put a flower on the grave. Known as 'Bird' by her sister, Ethel was called 'Garnie' by her grandchildren. Other regular visitors to Dunningwell included an aunt known as 'the Boozalier' who ineffectually disguised her brandy breath with eau-de-Cologne before going down to dinner.

Ethel always had breakfast in bed when she was at Dunningwell and her two young grandsons would go in to her bedroom to say good morning and share a portion of her boiled egg. She now had more time to spare for her grandsons than she had ever managed to find for their father. She would be sitting up with a shawl around her shoulders and her hair lying flat, but during the day her hair was set in a pair of winged pads, known as 'rats', and she enjoyed her grandsons' constant teasing about 'the rats escaping to frighten the maids'. She would chuckle affectionately, no matter how often this witticism was repeated. Her grandson observed how Ethel got on well with the servants because she never patronised them, never treated them like furniture or ignored them; her only malice being against 'vulgarians, bureaucrats and those jumped-up jacks in office'. She continued to indulge in good quality clothes and would think nothing of paying 20 guineas for a hat at a time when working men were earning around 30 shillings a week.

With Ethel and her husband leading separate lives, the grandchildren only saw their grandfather, who they fondly called 'Punda', once or twice a year at his London home in Cambridge Gate, where he lived contentedly with a Miss Percy.

In 1926, Ethel Fenwick founded the British College of Nurses. It was intended to be an educational body, in opposition to the College of Nursing Ltd, of whose conditions and aims she did not approve. She had not lost her fire with age, would not adjust her ideals and had little experience of accommodating any opposition. By this time, she had moved out of Wimpole Street and was living in a small eighteenth-century house in Barton Street, Westminster, surrounded by her priceless collection of antiques. She took a keen interest in politics and had always been a strong supporter of Winston Churchill, even during his 'wilderness years' between 1929 and 1939 when he had been ostracised by the Conservative Party for his outspoken opinions towards Free Trade, Irish Home Rule, and India.

When the next election for the GNC took place in 1927, Ethel Fenwick did not stand. She knew she would not have enough support to beat the College of Nursing candidates and wrote angrily, 'the majority of nurses in this kingdom are too ignorant of the true condition of nursing politics, and too subject to economic control, and to financial patronage, to give a free vote for candidates' (*British Journal of Nursing* editorial, November 1927).

Ethel had not lost her enthusiasm for travel, and in 1927 she attended an interim conference of the ICN in Geneva. The following year, 1928, she went to Rome for an international reunion of nurses, as part of the International Union against Tuberculosis. While in Rome she was presented to Mussolini, head of the Italian government, and she had an audience with the Pope. She also visited the villa where Florence Nightingale was born. That must have been a very special occasion for Ethel as, in spite of their differences of opinion on some matters, she had always been a great admirer of the influential Florence and of her undoubted organising abilities. On her return to England, Ethel was taken ill, confined to bed for six months and so was unable to attend the

ICN meeting in Montreal in 1929. It would be ten years before the ICN members could meet again at another Congress.

The first talking film *The Jazz Singer*, starring Al Jolson, thrilled audiences in 1927. In London, fourteen people died and the Westminster vaults were flooded as the Thames burst its banks following a combination of high tide and a thaw in 1928. In that year, the voting age for women was lowered from 30 to 21 and women were at last on an equal footing with male voters. It had been a long hard fight since women's suffrage was advocated by Mary Wollstonecraft in 1792.

Areas of unrest persisted throughout the world. Russia and China were in dispute over a jointly operated railway in Manchuria and there were Arab riots in Jerusalem. Chinese warlords competed for power while civil war and a strong anti-foreigner movement raged throughout the country. Chiang Kai-shek succeeded as leader of the China People's Party in 1928.

The French Premier, Aristotle Briand, proposed the creation of a United States of Europe but this idea for promotion of peace was not greeted with any enthusiasm. In 1928, the beginning of the American Wall Street Crash, in which thousands of accounts were suddenly wiped out, created unbelievable hardship and chaos.

In 1928, at the University of London School of Medicine, Alexander Fleming accidentally discovered penicillin. He attempted to isolate it for medical use, but was hampered by lack of expertise and equipment and it was to be many years before it became developed as an antibiotic. Ramsay MacDonald was once again Prime Minister and by 1929 Margaret Bradfield, a Trade Union leader, became the first woman appointed to a Cabinet position when she became Ramsay MacDonald's Minister of Labour.

Law enforcement had become an increasingly serious problem in America, thanks to the prohibition of alcohol and the gangland crime this engendered. In the 1929 St Valentine's Day massacre, seven of George 'Bugs' Moran's gangsters were killed by Al Capone's mobsters and half the Chicago police force were under investigation for corruption.

Flappers, the Charleston dance, long cigarette holders, feathered headgear, cloche hats, strings of pearls and beaded evening dresses were all the rage in the west. The *British Medical Journal* cautioned against silk stockings in cold weather as this modern fashion could cause erythema, chaffing and puffiness of the skin due to the 'scanty' covering of legs. This dire warning proved ineffective in changing the new fashions. Of more immediate concern to the British public was the sartorial rebellion by the United States Ambassador, who refused to wear traditional silk knee breeches at the court when he went to a Buckingham Palace reception. Even at a time when Coco Chanel was at the peak of her fashion-designing career, the Ambassador's revolt was seen in some quarters as an outrageous threat to tradition.

In October 1929, in the financial centre of America on Wall Street, stock prices collapsed, resulting in bankruptcy and hardship for many people.

At a time when the teaching of evolution was banned in the state of Tennessee and teacher John T. Scopes had been fined $100 for ignoring this edict, the Museum of National History was sponsoring an expedition to search for the earliest human origins in Outer Mongolia. By 1930, deaths in America due to alcoholism had risen six-fold since the introduction of prohibition and cigarette smoking soared.

In India, Gandhi began his peace march, campaigning for the end to British rule and the end to the British monopoly of salt tax. He was eventually arrested for causing civil unrest. In Britain there were 2.5 million unemployed and the economy went into crisis. Prime Minister Ramsay MacDonald offered his resignation in 1931, but remained in office as head of a coalition. The British Empire changed character in 1931 as Canada, Australia, New Zealand, South Africa and Newfoundland all become self-governing dominions, having equal status with Britain as members of British Commonwealth of Nations.

Exposure of legs remained a problem and in 1931 it was still possible to be fined 40/- for permitting a woman, presumably cleaning windows, to stand precariously on a windowsill.

In Scotland in 1931, the 12,000 Royal Navy sailors on fifteen Atlantic Fleet ships anchored in the deep waters at Invergordon in the Moray Firth went on strike in protest over servicemen's pay cuts – an incident which was not widely publicised at the time by the British newspapers.

While the worldwide economic depression deepened, unemployment figures reached historic levels and in Germany over five million people were without jobs. There were riots in London in protest against the high unemployment in Britain.

Despite previous imprisonment for his various protests against British rule, in November 1931, Mahatma Gandhi was invited to Buckingham Palace to meet India's Emperor George V and Queen Mary at a party for 500 guests. Conversation was stiffly polite, the subject being the English weather. In December the British–Indian peace talks broke down. By 1932, the Indian Congress party was outlawed and Gandhi was jailed for urging civil disorder at a time when peaceful picketing was declared illegal.

In June 1932, Amelia Earhart became the first woman to fly solo across the Atlantic, 'for the fun of it' in 14 hours, 16 minutes. Trouble continued as the jobless rioted in London and hunger marches took place throughout the country. Meanwhile, in 1932 at Cambridge University, the atom was split by Dr J. D. Cockroft and Dr E. T. S Walton. Their process released 60 per cent greater energy than the amount used, causing Lord Rutherford, the first man to split the atom in 1919, to acknowledge that, for the first time, more energy had been given out than was put into the process. Of more immediate relevance to the man in the street was the invention of the windproof and easy to use Zippo cigarette lighter.

In 1933, war clouds were clearly looming throughout the world. There was rioting in Spain as revolution spread and, after being criticised over its dispute with China, Japan walked out of the League of Nations. By January, as Hitler became Chancellor, Germany was on the brink of civil war. Fire gutted the Reichstag building and Hitler linked the incident to communist insurgency, persuading President von Hindenburg to grant emergency powers banning free speech and the right to protest. The German parliament was adjourned and Hitler became dictator. By March 1933, the Nazis had opened their first concentration camp, ten miles outside Munich, at a place called Dachau. Nazis burned books and embarked on their anti-communist and anti-trade union campaign and, in July, began their programme to purify the Aryan race.

By November 1933, over 22 million people had been to see the Chicago World Fair, which closed for the winter and reopened the following June. After years of chaos, criminality and mayhem, prohibition of alcohol was finally ended in America. The science of nutrition and its role in diseases of the body was developing rapidly and the 1934 Nobel prize in medicine was awarded to G. Minot and G. Whipple, who had discovered that the ingestion of beef liver was a successful treatment for pernicious anaemia.

Following the onslaught of a polio epidemic, many lives were saved with the aid of a brilliantly innovative machine designed by a Scotsman. Dr Robert Henderson, born in Clatt, Aberdeenshire, developed Britain's first iron lung in 1934 with the help of the Aberdeen City hospital's engineer. Having bought materials from local firms, including porthole scuttles and other objects from ships' chandlers, the two men cobbled it all together to create the machine which saved the life of a 10-year-old polio sufferer.

Despite this success, the bureaucrats quibbled and Dr Henderson was disciplined for unauthorised use of hospital facilities when building this life-saving iron lung. However, in 1939, Lord Nuffield, motor manufacturer and philanthropist, supplied 1,700 of these machines free of charge to hospitals in Britain and throughout the Empire – donating seventy-five to Scotland alone. Eventually, after saving hundreds of lives, the old 'lung' was replaced in the 1950s by pressure ventilators.

Having previously been appointed chairman of a British memorial committee, Ethel Fenwick was at last, in 1934, able to inaugurate the Florence Nightingale International Foundation. Encouraging nursing links, she was able to persuade her daughter-in-law to take bricks from

Florence Nightingale's home to various Canadian hospitals. These gifts were much appreciated and learning of their warm reception, Ethel proudly announced, 'Even my minions are treated with honour, appreciated abroad if not at home!'

Extremist ideology was on the rise but Sir Oswald Mosley and his Black Shirts had badly misjudged the mood of the British public when speaking at Olympia in 1934 and were surprised at their hostile reception. Britain found it necessary to increase defence spending to counter the growing possibility of a German threat. Prime Minister Stanley Baldwin was forced to acknowledge that the attempt to lead the world in unilateral disarmament had failed. Trouble was brewing in China, Nazi oppression continued in Germany, and Italian conflict raged in Ethiopia. Massive dust storms created havoc across enormous areas of America, destroying crops and forcing people to flee their homes. While Malcolm Campbell exceeded 300mph on the flats of Utah, and Howard Hughes set the aviation speed record of 351mph, Charles Lindenberg and Nobel prize winning scientist Alex Carrel created an artificial heart at the Rockefeller Institute. Their device managed to maintain organs alive in the laboratory for days and even weeks.

In 1935, twenty-five years after his coronation, George V and his wife, Queen Mary (May of Teck) reached their Silver Jubilee and the occasion was celebrated throughout the country. Ethel Fenwick held a strong dislike of Queen Mary, partly due to the Queen's animosity over many years towards her friend Princess Christian but also, it was suspected by the family, due to the Queen beating her to the prize on some antique hunt. At the time of the Jubilee, Ethel's grandson found it strange to hear his beloved 'Garnie' decrying 'that May of Teck'.

George V did not live long after his jubilee. He died in January 1936, aged 70, to be succeeded by Edward VIII. The Spanish Civil War erupted as General Francisco Franco led army forces in revolt against the Spanish government and many young British men volunteered to fight for freedom in Spain in support of their beliefs.

People and politicians protested, but no action was taken when the Nazis entered the Rhineland. In a futile attempt to draw attention to the plight of Jews in Germany, a 48-year-old Jewish man, Stefan Fox, shot himself during a League of Nations session. During the Berlin Olympics, American athlete Jesse Owens gave a brilliant performance. Irritated at his 'master race' being so humiliated by a black man, Hitler used the rain as excuse for not staying to offer his congratulations.

Britain was a troubled nation with an increasingly desperate number of unemployed men. In Jarrow, unemployment ran at 68 per cent and in October 1936, 200 jobless men marched to London with a petition. These Jarrow marchers were supported in a pre-march service by their MP, Miss Ellen Wilkinson.

Although Americans were aware of a constitutional crisis facing the British monarchy and were following events with interest, press baron Lord Beaverbrook enforced a news blackout. This ensured that the British public was kept in the dark about their future monarch's affair with a divorcee. Thanks to their compliant and subservient press, the British public were taken by surprise when, in December, the uncrowned Edward VIII went into exile with Wallis Simpson and was succeeded by his brother, George VI. The following year, 1937, George VI was crowned, with his mother, the widowed Queen Mother, May of Teck, demonstrating her full support at the ceremony. Edward and Wallis Simpson were married in France, never permitted to set foot on English soil again.

In Russia the Stalinist purges increased; Guernica, capital of the Basque Country, was strafed by German bombers in 1937, and the Japanese-Chinese skirmishes intensified with the Japanese bombing of Shanghai. Rivals Chiang Kai-shek and Mao Tse-tung were united against the Japanese enemy. The United States became unwittingly involved when, in December, the Japanese sank United States ships after mistaking them for Chinese vessels.

A massive Nazi rally at Nuremberg was a spectacular success but, the following month in London, Oswald Mosley experienced no such triumph. Despite some powerful backers, when hoping to emulate his hero he was showered with stones instead of adulation.

Meanwhile, a revolutionary new thread had been developed by American chemist Wallace Hume Carothers. Commercial production of this synthetic polymer fibre, nylon, begun in 1938, was to have a major world impact and laid the foundation of the synthetic-fibre industry. Sadly, Carothers suffered from depression and committed suicide in 1937 before the full impact of his invention had been appreciated. Within a year, highly prized nylon stockings were on sale and developments had begun into the uses of nylon within medicine and surgery.

The 1938 Nobel prize was awarded to a physicist, Professor Enrico Fermi, who had fled to the United States from fascist Rome a year previously. He achieved the prize for his vital work on radioactivity. Still safely in supervised care, Typhoid Mary died six years after suffering a stroke. No one knew just how many deaths she had been responsible for during her catering career.

Ethel Fenwick's final campaign was fought over the issue of a second grade of nurse. The 1905 Select Committee on Registration had foreseen that one likely consequence of a three-year training would be a shortage of candidates entering the profession. The committee had advised that it might be necessary to consider a separate register of a lower standard. Ethel Fenwick disagreed, believing that the supply of educated intelligent girls was sufficient, asserting that it was simply a case of attracting them to the profession.

After the First World War, the increases in career choices open to women contributed to a shortage of nurses in the 1920s and 1930s. It is interesting to note that by 1937 only 120 men were in nurse training. The shortage was so acute that smaller voluntary hospitals and infirmaries advertised for, and employed, assistant nurses. These were women who did not wish to undertake training, or girls who had been rejected by training schools. The numbers of assistant nurses were so large that, by 1936, their unofficial status could no longer be ignored and the College of Nursing recommended their enrolment, on a separate roll to be set up by the General Nursing Council. The BMA came out in support of recognition in 1937 and that same year the government committee, under the chairmanship of Lord Athlone, made similar recommendations to those of the College.

The Royal British Nurses' Association and the British College of Nurses as well as the *British Journal of Nursing* protested against this perceived threat to the trained nurse. Having spent best part of her life fighting to establish the professional status of nursing based on a qualification consisting of three years training, Ethel Fenwick defended that standard to the last:

> We shall fight this proposal to the death. It is 62 years since I entered a hospital for training. During the fight for the Registration Bill I practically lived in the lobbies of the Houses of Parliament. We won, and it cost us between £20,000 and £30,000. But this proposal to give professional status to unqualified nurses would destroy everything we worked for, and we won't have it.
> 
> (*The Evening Standard*, 18 March 1939)

Not one to settle for a quiescent old age, Ethel organised a public meeting in Caxton Hall, Westminster to protest, and published a pamphlet, 'A Demand for Justice for the State Registered Nurse'. However, in May the GNC accepted the necessity of recognising a second grade of nurse, a decision which was accelerated by the outbreak of the Second World War. The Civil Nursing Reserve, responsible for the recruitment of nurses during the war, accepted assistant nurses from the start.

At this time, Ethel Fenwick was still living in the little house in Barton Street. Her home was packed with porcelain, Rockingham and Staffordshire miniature animals, journeyman's pieces, face screens in lacquer and mother-of-pearl, Chinese porcelain, fine mahogany furniture, and a collection of miniature family portraits. She collected Regency and Victorian furniture when it was out of fashion as well as many more items that took her fancy. She encouraged her grandson

David to take an interest in antiques and always gave him something to take away whenever he visited his beloved 'Garnie'.

By 1939, war was inevitable, in spite of Neville Chamberlain's attempt to appease Hitler and announcing 'peace in our time'. In Germany, Nazis burned 267 synagogues and destroyed thousands of Jewish homes and businesses – the violent smashing of windows gave the night its name of '*Kristallnacht*'. In April 1939, all German children were ordered to serve in the Hitler Youth Organisation.

Notions of racial supremacy and intolerance also flourished outside Nazi Germany. In early 1939, the hitherto respected organisation Daughters of the American Revolution refused to allow the black American contralto, Marian Anderson, to sing at the Constitution Hall, Washington. Outraged, the First Lady, Eleanor Roosevelt, resigned from the organisation. The conductor Artoo Toscanini, who had previously fled to America from Nazi persecution, believed the singer's voice was one that came once in 100 years. Together with Mrs Roosevelt, he arranged for the singer to perform at an outdoor concert.

Meantime, also fleeing Nazi persecution, over 900 Jewish refugees were refused permission to land in the safe haven of Cuba from the liner *St Louis*. Permission to land was also refused from America and Canada; the ship returned to Europe with the refugees where Britain, Belgium, the Netherlands, and France each accepted a proportion of the refugees. Many of those who landed in Europe were later caught by the Nazis and 254 of them were murdered during the Holocaust.

The two-year long World Fair was opened in Flushing Meadows, New York in 1939 and contained exhibitions from sixty nations. Newly developed nylon and cellophane were shown to over a million of the visitors, nylon stockings by then being more desirable and cheaper than silk. In June 1939, British royalty, King George and Queen Elizabeth, visited this spectacular exhibition, much to the delight of the American public.

Ethel had more to think about than the war when her husband, Dr Bedford Fenwick, died in October 1939. Until his retirement, he had been physician to the Hospital for Women, Soho Square, as well as a Royal Gynaecologist, and a distinguished Wimpole Street specialist. Although they had lived in separate establishments for many years and had a tempestuous relationship, Dr Bedford Fenwick had always been a staunch supporter of Ethel and a firm ally in her lengthy struggles for registration. Together they had achieved much, not the least being their son Christian, who had fought and been wounded in the First World War and was now a county court judge. His son David, then at Cambridge University, helped his mother clear the personal effects from Dr Bedford Fenwick's home at Cambridge Gate, where he had been living for years with Miss Percy.

It was prudent for the doctor's daughter-in-law and grandson to deal with this sensitive situation and Miss Percy remained hovering around while the clearing operation took place. It was thought important that many private and personal documents, papers, and letters should be discreetly burnt – they doubtless contained much interesting medical and social information, now sadly lost. Miss Percy was quite vehement in her antagonism towards Ethel during the clearout but David was able to take away and treasure the Vienna china ornament which he had been told that grateful patient, Lillie Langtry, had given his grandfather.

It was discovered that Dr Bedford Fenwick's sense of responsibility and protective support had extended beyond the feisty Ethel. In order to shield his two sisters from the knowledge that a disastrous investment in the railways had depleted their savings, he and his family had discreetly supported these genteel unmarried ladies for many years.

Ethel Fenwick gave up her own flat when the war began and moved into a smaller flat on top of the British College of Nurses premises in Portland Place. However, the College moved and the Portland Place quarters were given up early in the war. From then on Ethel, now in her eighties, lived in accommodation at the headquarters of the RBNA in Queen's Gate, Kensington, from where she continued to take an active interest in nursing affairs.

In September 1940, the London Blitz began. Over 7,000 people were killed and around 9,000 were injured with many being made homeless and having to sleep in the underground railway stations. Water mains were severed initially by parachute mines and then over 10,000 firebombs were dropped. Fires raged out of control. Twenty thousand firemen were reinforced by soldiers and civilians. Many of them were killed in the process of fighting the fires amongst the unstable collapsing buildings and rubble. Fire-watching duties were tightened up, and it was made compulsory for all eligible civilians, male and female, to do their share of fire-watch duty as well as their normal employment. Fines of £100 or three months' imprisonment were handed out to shirkers.

Once again, British women helped out in the manpower shortage. Much of the essential work they undertook would have been unimaginable or non-existent in Ethel's youth – varying from radio operators, drivers, ambulance drivers, aviators, and land girls. The Minister of Labour, Ernest Bevin, called for women to come forward to fill vital jobs, such as those in shell factories. Child-minding facilities, as well as day and night nurseries, were provided to enable women to take up vital employment. Many women and girls were employed within the armed forces where new provisions had to be arranged for them and their requirements catered for. Lord Nuffield donated sanitary towels for the use of the forces' female personnel, many of whom, familiar only with washing out and reusing cloths and old rags, had never seen such modern items before. Apparently these modern 'bunnies', 'Nuffies' or 'Lord Nuffields' made an excellent job of shining uniform shoes!

The scientists worked hard to improve weapons technology and, in 1941, the first controlled nuclear chain reaction opened the way to atomic bombs and nuclear energy.

Ethel Fenwick took a lively interest in the progress of the war and was incensed by news reports of the bad treatment of nurses captured in the Far East. While in Queens Gate she discovered that interned diplomats were being exercised daily in Kensington Gardens. Outraged, she altered her whole regime in order to force a confrontation. Ignoring the protective police escort, she would angrily prod the hapless diplomats with her umbrella. On more than one occasion, she charged and scattered them while raging about the disgraceful government which allowed the Royal Gardens to be defiled. She was bitterly disappointed when they refused to prosecute her for assault. Instead, a decision was taken to go elsewhere to exercise and the irate old lady was unable to embarrass them further!

In spite of the war, or perhaps because of it, people made good use of their free time. The jitterbug became all the rage, the days of chaperones and society balls were long gone and people from all walks of life found themselves mixing together. Talent and qualifications were far more important than social status as the exigencies of the times broke through many class barriers.

In December 1942, the Beveridge report proposed the creation of a Welfare State which would offer security from the cradle to the grave, envisaging full and free hospital care for everyone, along with state retirement pensions. Then, in 1943, the Minister of Health introduced a Nurses Bill to enable the General Nursing Council to set up a roll of assistant nurses. Proving that she most certainly was not in her dotage, Ethel Fenwick wrote to the Prime Minister, Winston Churchill, to protest. In an editorial, 'The Rise and Decline of the Profession of Nursing', she compared the proposed legislation to the registration of 'quack' doctors, considering the dreadful prospect that nursing as a profession for educated women might cease to exist. At the age of 86, she returned to the lobbies of the House of Commons, her last hope of support. However, the Nurses Act became law on 22 April 1943.

The war raged on. The 18-year-old Princess Elizabeth showed the country that she could 'do her bit' for the war effort, and became a junior subaltern in the women's services, learning the skills of a proficient auto mechanic. When the first of the V1 rocket bombs fell on London, women and children were evacuated to safer places in the countryside and the royal family slept each night at Windsor Castle. By July, 2,752 people had been killed by the V1 bombs, and more terror followed as the silent V2 bombs hit London in September.

Ethel's sister Clara had married young and had refused to have children with her long-suffering husband, but she had been devastated when he died suddenly in 1910. Her later years had been somewhat lonely with only occasional visitors and her cook, maid, and two gardeners to keep her company. One of the duties of the maid was to look out of the window to check and report who was at the door and Clara would then instruct her to open the door – or not – as she decreed. Since being widowed, Clara had always worn black, her clothes becoming older and more worn and faded with the passing years. With no form of private transport and with only one car in the village, she became quite isolated in her old age.

Clara died aged 90, at Dunningwell, as the war was drawing to a close, and after her death her effects were cleared up by her nephew Christian. Amongst her documents and letters, he discovered many referring to a local scandal involving a woman known only as the 'Ollie Bird'. The documents and letters were all burnt and any stories remain forever lost. The estate was sold and the elderly maid was obliged to go into the workhouse at Workington.

Eventually the tide of war turned and in 1945 the prison camp of Auschwitz was liberated. Scenes of horror were being discovered there and in the other massive Nazi death camps. In America, on the eve of victory, President Roosevelt died of a cerebral haemorrhage and Harry Truman assumed the presidency. Mussolini was shot and hanged, and Hitler committed suicide in his bunker. At last, the Germans surrendered unconditionally and huge crowds celebrated VE day in London. On 26 June 1945, a United Nations charter was created to establish world peace.

Stories from the concentration camps of Germany begin to filter through. Surviving prisoners of war revealed conditions of their prison camps and of the horrific forced marches they had endured across Europe during one of the coldest recorded winters in recent European history. These reports, along with others from the Far East of beatings, forced marches, starvation and torture caused shock and outrage as the public become aware of the torture and suffering endured by soldiers and civilians. In August 1945, atomic bombing forced the Japanese to surrender and in January 1946 a shamed Emperor Hirohito stunned his entire nation when he solemnly declared his assumed divinity, implicitly believed by his subjects, to be nothing but a myth. The Nuremberg trials of war criminals began in November. Any sense of triumph in victory was muted by the realisation of mankind's capability for cruelty.

With high hopes of preventing another world war, the first session of the United Nations General Assembly took place in January 1946, at the Methodist Central Hall, London. In July 1946, the first nuclear bomb was tested at Bikini Atoll and controversy about the moral issue of such a weapon began to emerge. In October 1946, Nazi war criminals were hanged and, it was hoped, so ending one shameful episode in world history.

Thanks to the work and nutritional advice of Lord John Boyd Orr (founder of the Rowatt Institute, and eventual Nobel peace prize winner), the wartime diet of the nation had resulted in many people being far healthier than they had been during the 1930's. Lord Boyd Orr became Director-General of the Food and Agricultural Organisation of the newly formed United Nations, but later resigned when his advice was not implemented. Some experts believed problems of world famine would now be less severe had his advice been followed.

Ethel Fenwick followed the world news as keenly as ever. Age had not mellowed her, and her opinions about the treatment of imprisoned Allied troops, and especially the mistreatment of nurses, were outspoken and uncompromising in their condemnation. She was now approaching her 90th year but was still working, actively participating in production of her nursing journal. One day in June 1946, as she was leaving the College of Nursing building, she fell and fractured her femur. She was given a private room in St Bartholomew's hospital and treated with great care by her devoted nurses.

Sadly, the fracture never healed, presumably due to a degree of osteoporosis due to her age. In November she was transferred to the home of a friend, the wife of the vicar of Colney Hatch, London, who described what followed:

> For some time she appeared to rally, and once more interested herself in Nursing affairs ... Her 90th birthday came round on January 26th, and she received many little tokens, and cables from friends abroad ... but her rally was short-lived and gradually she became weaker ... became unconscious on March 10th and never recovered. She died on the evening of March 13th at 10.30pm and at long last that courageous and indomitable spirit found rest.
> (*British Journal of Nursing*, April 1947, p. 42)

Her father had been buried in the little graveyard at Spynie, near the ruins of the old palace and, not many yards away, the ashes of Ramsay MacDonald had been interred. However, widespread floods, following a severe winter, prevented Ethel's body being taken north to the family burial ground. Her remains were cremated at Golders Green on 18 March, where twenty-eight years earlier her rival and opponent Eva Luckes had been buried. The next day a memorial service was held at St Bartholomew's hospital. Ethel had been an honorary member of the national nurse associations of America, Germany, Finland, and India and fulsome tributes to her work came from all over the international nursing world.

In May 1947, the *British Journal of Nursing* reported the ceremony that took place on 9 April 1947 when Ethel Fenwick's ashes were interred in the precincts of Thoroton Church.

> The last journey of her earthly remains lay through the lanes, highways and quaint villages of the beautiful Trent Valley ... the familiar scene of her earliest years.

Ethel's childhood home, Thoroton Hall, was just visible through the trees as sweet violets were dropped in her grave. Her last resting place is marked with these inscriptions: 'She raised the status of the nursing profession and secured its recognition by Parliament' and 'I have fought a good fight'.

The funeral had been privately arranged by her only son, Christian, and his family. In the church at Thoroton is a stained-glass window depicting St Agnes, the patron saint of nurses, with the inscription: 'In memory of George Storer their stepfather and Harriette his wife, this window was erected by her children, Clara, Ethel and Eric, 1909.'

Two months after Ethel's death, in May 1947, the International Nursing Congress met in Atlantic City where it had been intended to present their founder with a citation in recognition of her 'unique and life-long contribution to the advancement of nursing profession throughout the world'.

The National Health Service came into being in 1948 and, thanks to Ethel Fenwick's lengthy campaigns, registered nurses were ready to take their place beside the other professionals in caring for the health of the nation. Some have sacrificed their lives for their patients, not least the hundreds who have died while caring for patients during the recent Covid-19 pandemic. Ethel cared deeply about her nurses and ensured their profession was one to be respected. In doing so, she left the world of nursing in a much better state than she had found it.

# Acknowledgements

The instigator of the original book (*The First Nurse: Ethel Bedford Fenwick*, Librario, 2003) was the late Mary Thorogood – District Nursing Officer Grampian Health Board West District, BA (Open University), RGN, SCM, Nursing Administration Hospital Certificate, elected member of the RCN Scottish Board, elected member GNC Scotland, Member of the Disciplinary Committee, Member of the Scottish Matrons' Association, and their representative on Nursing and Midwifery on the Whitley Council.

Mary became interested in Ethel's story when, living in Elgin, Moray, she read a brief resume of Ethel's career in the League of St Bartholomew's booklet and realised that this unsung innovator was born in Moray. After obtaining more information through her old nursing colleagues at Barts, she suggested I compose a pamphlet or booklet to be available in the local Elgin Museum. But Ethel's life could not be easily condensed and, instead of a list of dates and committees, the focus widened to include subjects and world events that affected Ethel's long and eventful life.

Many years later, I was contacted by an enthusiastic Liz Howard-Thornton and with her encouragement, fewer distractions, a renewed sense of purpose, and some new information, the book has been revised and rewritten. Hopefully, for the centenary of the opening of the Nurse's Register, it will provide a better general understanding of the remarkable Ethel and her campaigns, as well as providing an insight into her life and times.

First and foremost, without the work and research done by Winifred Hector, M.Phil., SRN, SCM, DN (Univ. of London), RNT, Lecturer

Queen Elizabeth College, University of London, and Principal Tutor at St Bartholomew's Hospital, none of this work would have been possible. Sincere thanks are due to her for giving permission to quote freely from her book, *The Work of Mrs Bedford Fenwick and the Rise of Professional Nursing* (Whitefriars Press, 1973), based on a thesis she presented in 1970, and her history of *The Royal Hospital of Saint Bartholomew's*.

Another valuable source of information was *The Battle of the Nurses* (Scutari Press, 1992), by Susan McGann, who also gave permission to borrow from her work on Ethel Bedford Fenwick.

The late David Fenwick, grandson of Ethel Fenwick, gave me information and encouragement to go ahead with the original project and was kind enough to give his permission to quote freely from his reminiscences – although some discretion has been used!

Thanks are due to the London NHS Trust and Marion Rea, Archivist, St Bartholomew's for her help. I am also grateful for much information and encouragement from Catherine Clarke, Val Wood, John O'Reilly, the committee of the Ethel Gordon Fenwick commemorative Partnership, and the ever-supportive Liz Howard-Thornton.

Many thanks also to A. B. Loveland for his very patient support and help with the photographs.

Elgin, 2021

# Sources

**Other sources of reference are:**

Baker, J., *Tolstoy's Bicycle*, Helicon 1995
Baren, M., *How it All Began*, Smith & Settle 1992
Castleden, R., *British History*, Paragon 1994
*Chronicle of the 20th Century*, Dorling Kindersley 1996
Eagle, R., *Seton Gordon, Life and Times of a Highland Gentleman*, Lochar Publishing Ltd 1991
*Encyclopedia Britannica*, 1997
Hudson, R., *The Jubilee Years*, compilation, Folio Society 1996
Johnson, B., *Steam Traction Engines, Wagons & Rollers*, Blanford 1976
Keay, J. & J., *Collins Encyclopedia of Scotland*, HarperCollins 1994
Magnusson, M., ed., *Chambers Biographical Dictionary*, Chambers 1990
Maunders, S., *The Treasury of History*, Ballantyne Hudson & Co 1876
Morgan, K., *The Oxford Illustrated History of Britain*, Oxford University Press 1995
Nader, R., *Canada Firsts*, M&S 1992
Reader's Digest, *Everyday Life Through the Ages* 1992
*The Definitive Edition of Rudyard Kipling's Verse*, Hodder & Stoughton 1945
*The Police Manual for Scotland*, prepared by a Committee of Chief Constables of Scotland, 7th edition, 1931, based on first edition, McCorquodale & Co 1893
Woodham Smith, C., *Queen Victoria*, BCA 1973
Yeo, G., *Nursing at Barts*, Alan Sutton 1995

# Index

Acland, Dr Henry, 75
Ambulance Association, 17
American Civil War, 6, 36
American Federation of Labour, 74
Anaesthetic, 35,
   pre-anaesthetics, 47
Anderson, Elizabeth Garret, 18, 22, 24, 26
Aspirin, 90
Asquith, Herbert, 127
Army nurses, 36–7
Assistant nurses, 170–71, 175

Barnardo, Thomas, 10
Barry, James, 9
Beeton, Isabella, 5
Bessant, Annie, 82–3
Beveridge report, 175
Bicycle, 67–8, 160
Blackwell, Elizabeth, 24
Blood transfusion, 133
Bly, Nellie, 64, 157
Bodichon, Barbara, 2, 26
Boer War, 17, 94, 98–9, 100, 107, 108, 109, 114
   concentration camps, 109
Bonham-Carter, Sir Henry, 84
Booth, William, 9, 15
Bowes Lyon, Elizabeth, 101, 158, 161
British College of Nurses, 163, 171, 173
British Medical Association, 80, 88, 108, 112, 115
British Nurses' Association, 75–6, 78
British Journal of Nursing, 76, 87, 110, 118, 135–6, 151, 155, 159, 163, 171, 178

British Red Cross Society, 135, 139
Burdett, Henry, 75, 79, 87, 89
Butler, Josephine, 21, 23, 26

Carrel, Dr Alexis, 129
Cavell, Edith, 137
Central Committee for Registration of Nurses, 159
Chartist movement, 4
Chicago World Fair, 84–6, 167
Churchill, Winston, 15, 100, 110, 126, 128, 163, 175
Civil Nursing Reserve, 171
College of Nursing, 139, 145, 147
Contagious Diseases Act, 26
Coronation, George V, 127
Crimea, 36
Curie, Marie, 94, 110, 114, 128

Darwin, Charles, 5
Davis, Emily, 24, 25
Davidson, Emily Wilding., 131
Dock, Lavina, 85–6, 96
Dunningwell, 16–17, 105–6, 117, 122, 148, 161–2

Edward VIII, 169
Electricity, 42
Electrocardiogram, 159

Factories Bill, 20
Fawcett, Henry, 18, 26
Fenwick, Dr Bedford, 41, 68–9, 122, 132, 138, 172–3
Fenwick, Christian, 78, 84, 173, 179
Fleming, Alexander, 164

Garret, Millicent, 17, 26
  Elizabeth 18, 22, 24, 36
General Nursing Council, 154, 155, 156, 159, 160, 163, 175
George V, 168
Girton College, for women, 12, 14
Gordon, 3
Gordon House Home Hospital, 74
Graeco-Turkish War, 89–90, 157
Gray, Josephine, 26
  *see also* Butler
Greenwich Mean Time, 41, 65

Hardie, Keir, 82, 83, 94, 116, 137
Hector, Winifred, 44, 46–8
Helsinki Congress 160
Henderson, Dr Robert, 167
Hesse, Angelina, 63, 113
Hill, Octavia, 9
Hitler, Adolf, 166, 176
Hobhouse, Emily, 107
Holland, Sydney, 121
Hospital Association, 75

Infection, 36–7, 58, 63, 159
Infectious Diseases (Notification) Act, 82
Influenza, 98, 145, 149
Iron Lung, 167
Inglis, Elsie, 64, 95, 110, 114, 134–5
Insulin, 154, 160
International Council of Women, 77, 86, 90, 95
International Nursing Congress, 86, 90, 116, 120, 128, 160
International Council of Nurses, 96–7, 103, 105, 110, 116, 120, 128, 160, 163, 179
International Council of Women, 77, 86, 95
International Women's Day, 127

Jex-Blake, Sophia, 26
Journalists, Society of Women, 127

Kaiser, 5, 91, 119, 126, 129
Koch, Robert, 63, 113

Lecture, by Ethel Manson, 60–62
Lister, Joseph, 11, 37, 109
Liston, Robert, 35
London Hospital, 40–42
  Bulletin, 43
London School of Medicine for Women, 26
Luckes, Eva, 41, 81, 84, 88, 107, 112, 121, 146–7, 178

Maas, Clara, 106
MacDonald, Ramsay, 3, 10, 128, 159, 164, 165, 178
Machin, Maria, 52–3
Male Nurses' Temperance Cooperation, 81
Mallon, Mary, *see* Typhoid Mary
Manchester Royal Infirmary, 39, 40, 
Manson, David, 1, 3, 178
Manson, Captain Eric, 4, 122, 139
Marmite, 102
Marriage, Clara, 16–17
  Ethel, 69, 71–2
Matron, duties of, 50–52,
Matron's Council, 88, 96, 107
Matron, Ethel appointed, 43, 53
  reforms, 53–7, 58–9
Medals, ix
Medical degrees for women, 26–7
Medical Register, 35, 36
Middlethorpe Hall, 13
Midwives Act, 107
Mill, John Stuart, 11, 23
Mussolini, 147, 157, 163, 176
Myers, Charles, 16, 125
  Clara, 176

National Health Service, 179
National Council of Trained Nurses of Great Britain and Ireland, 110
National Union of Women's Suffrage Society, 90, 118

# Index    185

Nazi Party, 158, 161, 169, 172, 177
Newspaper article, Miss Manson, 59–62
Nightingale, Florence, 5, 22, 35, 38, 79–80, 84, 87, 95, 108, 123, 128–9
  International Foundation, 167
Nottingham Children's Hospital, 38–9
  Ethel's interview, 38
Nurse Registration, 74, 76, 79, 107, 108, 112, 117–18, 125–6, 132, 133, 139, 146, 147, 149, 151
Nurses Registration Act, 150, 151
Nurse training, 28, 38, 49, 62
Nursing Record, 79, 81, 84, 87, 104, 110, 112
Nursing Mirror, 88

Orr, John Boyd, 158, 177
Overton, Lord, 94

Pageant of Women's Trades and Professions, 120
Paget, James, 47–8, 52, 70, 84
Panama Canal, 106
Pankhurst, Emmeline, 91, 109, 114, 119, 130
Pasteur, Louis, 37, 63, 64
Pavlov, Ivan, 111
Penicillin, 164
Pirie, Dr George Alexander, 94
Population changes, 13, 98
Princess Christian (Helena), 77–8, 154, 158
Probationers, 56, 58
  special probationers, 57, 58
Psychiatric care, 64, 82

Queen Victoria, 8, 17, 24, 35, 93, 104
  Golden Jubilee, 70
  Diamond Jubilee, 91–3

Red Cross, founding of, 6, 105, 123
Reed, Walter, 106
Reform Bill, 23, 63

Register of Nurses, 76, 125, 154
  *see also* nurse registration
Refrigeration, 48
Rontgen, Wilhelm, 64, 106
Royal British Nurses Association, 79, 88, 89, 108, 171
Royal Charter, 86–7
Rubber, 17
  gloves, 83
Russia, 111, 129, 142, 143, 144

Saint Bartholomew's Hospital, 43–6, 50–53, 55, 56, 149–150, 177
  early nurse training account, 28–33
  School of Nursing, 50
Saint Thomas's Hospital, Nursing school, 38, 49–50
Salvation Army, 15
Sanger, Margaret, 141
Scottish Women's Hospitals, 134–5
Scottish Women's Suffrage Federation, 114
Seacole, Mary, 36
Semmelweis, Ignaz, 37
Sewell, May Wright, 77, 86, 95
Simpson, James, 35
Smith, Dr Henry Louis, 94
Snow, John, 35
Society for the State Registration of Nurses, 107
Society of Women Journalists, 127
Spynie, 1–3, 4
Steam sterilisation, 65, 85
Stewart, Isla, 69, 75, 88, 123–4
Stockdale, Sister Henrietta, 78
Stopes, Marie, 41, 144, 153
Storer, George, 6–8, 12, 15, 64, 77
  against votes for women speech, 40
Storer, Harriet, 3, 7, 117
Stuart Mill, John, 11
Suffrage Bill, 4, 11, 14, 23, 113, 115, 133, 144, 164
  demonstrations, 118, 120, 127
Suffragettes, 115, 118, 129, 130, 131, 133
Swift, Sara, 139

Takamine, Jokichi, 108–9
Thoroton, 6, 16,
   Church, 178–9
   Hall, 7
Trained Nurses Institute, 87
Typhoid Mary, 111, 116, 125, 132, 170

University, women, 12, 14, 153

Voluntary Aid Detachments, 135

War, 1914–1918, 133, 135, 140–45
   Ethel's war work, 138

Welfare State, 127, 175
Wilkinson, Dr Matthew, 13, 39
   Fanny and Louisa, 17
Wollstonecraft, Mary, 4
Women's suffrage, 4, 11, 12, 14, 90, 115, 141
   Property Act, 12
   Bill, 24
Women in work, 20, 142, 174

X-rays, 64, 94, 106, 124